Foreword

A Victorian lady, moved, perhaps, by a sudden sense of transcendence due to over-tight corsetry, once proclaimed at a social gathering that she accepted the Universe. She has achieved immortality through Thomas Carlyle's atrabilious comment 'Gad, she'd better.' With like reason, we had better accept that the populations of the world are ageing. There is no thinkable alternative future, but politicians and planners seem unready to recognise the extent to which the structures, functions and priorities of ageing societies will have to change. It will surely be sensible for changes to be planned, rational and adaptive, rather than driven by short-term expediency or attempts to defend an unsustainable status quo.

In surveying growth in longevity from a range of viewpoints, this volume of presentations to the Royal College of Physicians testifies both to the pervasive nature of the adaptations required of an ageing society, and to the need to ensure their integration into coherent policy. We cannot evaluate health technologies, for example, without specifying what aims health technologies are expected to pursue. But are those aims expected to be prescribed by economists, defined by philosophers, or assumed by default? Whatever their provenance, such aims have to be set as dependable seamarks for a steadfast course through the changing winds of media interest and gale-force gusts from political lobbying.

The ageing of populations is a triumph of civilisation and an opportunity for a happier world, but the issues are too big for politics. Hope for the best future lies with sustained pressure from a concerned and informed legion of the public. To the members of that elite body the contributors to this book have consecrated their efforts.

JOHN GRIMLEY EVANS
Green College, Oxford

January 1998

Increasing lon

Medical, social and political implications

Edited by

Raymond Tallis

Professor of Geriatric Medicine, University of Manchester

1998

ROYAL COLLEGE OF PHYSICIANS
OF LONDON

Acknowledgements

I am grateful to the Royal College of Physicians for suggesting and hosting the meeting that formed the basis of this book and, in particular, Professor Humphrey Hodgson, lately Academic Registrar, who made the initial approach. I am also very grateful to Diana Beaven who saw that the meeting could form the basis of a book, ran with the idea and extracted manuscripts from speakers who, having spoken, imagined their duties were discharged. My gratitude extends, of course, to the speakers who responded generously to Diana's request for manuscripts. And finally I would like to record my debt to Amanda May for her tremendous support and for seeing the book through every stage of the production process.

RT

Royal College of Physicians of London
11 St Andrews Place, London NW1 4LE

Registered Charity No. 210508

Copyright © 1998 Royal College of Physicians of London
ISBN 1 86016 077 8

Typeset by Dan-Set Graphics, Telford, Shropshire
Printed in Great Britain by Sarum Print Limited, Salisbury, Wiltshire

British Library Cataloguing in Publication Data
A catalogue record of this book is available from the British Library

Contributors

Professor Shah Ebrahim *Professor of Clinical Epidemiology, Royal Free Hospital School of Medicine, Department of Primary Care and Population Sciences, Rowland Hill Street, London NW3 2PF*

Professor Sir John Grimley Evans *Professor of Clinical Geratology, The Radcliffe Infirmary, Woodstock Road, Oxford OX2 6HE*

Dr Emily Grundy *Reader in Social Gerontology, Centre for Population Studies, London School of Hygiene and Tropical Medicine, Keppel Street, London WC1E 7HT*

Professor Chris Ham *Professor of Health Policy and Management and Director of the Health Services Management Centre, University of Birmingham, 40 Edgbaston Park Road, Birmingham B15 2RT*

Professor John Harris *Sir David Alliance Professor of Bioethics and Director, Institute for Medicine, Law and Bioethics, Humanities Building, University of Manchester, Oxford Road, Manchester M13 9PL*

Professor Michael A Horan *Professor of Geriatric Medicine, Department of Geriatric Medicine, Clinical Gerontology Group, Clinical Sciences Building, Hope Hospital, Salford M6 8HD*

Professor Sir Miles Irving *Director of the NHS Health Technology Programme and Professor of Surgery, Department of Surgery, University of Manchester, Hope Hospital, Clinical Sciences Building, Salford M6 8HD*

Professor Malcolm L Johnson *Professor of Health and Social Policy, Director, School for Policy Studies, University of Bristol, Rodney Lodge, Grange Road, Bristol BS8 4EA*

Dr Alexandre Kalache *Chief, Ageing and Health Programme, World Health Organization, 1211 Geneva 27, Switzerland*

Ms Ingrid Keller *Programme Assistant, Ageing and Health Programme, World Health Organization, 1211 Geneva 27, Switzerland*

Professor Thomas B L Kirkwood *Professor of Biological Gerontology, Biological Gerontology Group, Department of Geriatric Medicine and School of Biological Sciences, University of Manchester, 3.239 Stopford Building, Oxford Road, Manchester M13 9PT*

Professor Alan Maynard *Professor of Health Economics, York Health Economics Consortium, University of York, Heslington, York YO1 5DD*

Professor Anthony M Warnes *Professor of Social Gerontology, Centre for Ageing and Rehabilitation Studies, University of Sheffield, Community Sciences Centre, Northern General Hospital, Herries Road, Sheffield S5 7AU*

Editor's introduction

One of the most profound, and certainly the most enduring of the many revolutions of the last few centuries, has been the ageing of the world's population. Two thirds of mankind's improvement in longevity has occured in this century and, for the first time in history, most middle-aged citizens in some first world countries have more grandparents than children. Moreover, there has been a sharp rise – set to continue for many decades – in the numbers of the very aged. In the UK, the over 85s have increased more than five-fold since 1950, and the Queen sends out ten times as many congratulatory telegrams to centenarians than she did when she came to the throne.

Perversely, this triumph, which has many causes – the application of technology to meeting physiological needs and ensuring physical safety, social welfare policies, public health measures and, more specifically, scientific medicine – has been read by some commentators as a disaster. There is much negative hyperbole about the economic threat of non-productive elders with their burdensome pensions and, more important, their revenue-consuming illnesses and disabilities. The latter have prompted much anxious speculation and it has even been suggested, as in Roy Porter's recent authoritative history of medicine,[1] that medicine is now facing a crisis in its sense of purpose, with 'the law of diminishing returns' applying to the use of medical resources to improve health and prolong life. 'What an ignominious destiny', Porter reflects, 'if the future of medicine turns into bestowing meagre increments of unenjoyed life!'[2]

The view that added years have been, or will be, bought only at the cost of added distress is at odds with some of the most recent findings emerging from longitudinal studies[3]. Although the picture is not entirely clear, the data increasingly suggest that the period of disability before death is shrinking despite an increased life-span; that there is a 'compression of morbidity'[4]. While this is not being achieved with the speed anticipated by Fries and Crapo in their seminal paper, modest optimism seems to have better justification than panic.

Further improvements in the health, independence and life chances of older people will not occur spontaneously. Increasing medical expertise, improved attitudes within the medical profession and in society at large and, partly as a reflection of this, a more generous allocation of resources will be essential to ensure that better medical treatments are delivered in a more user-friendly and equitable way. Health care, however, goes beyond the delivery of treatments narrowly construed; it encompasses health promotion and preventive medicine. And although health is one of the major determinants of well-being in old age, there are other important influences. These include tangible elements such as economic status and intangible ones such as the attitudes of others which translate, when internalised, into a sense of who, what and why one is. Low self-esteem resulting from marginalisation may have as important an adverse effect on quality of life in old age as poor health.

An unprejudiced, non-hysterical and numerate debate about the implications of increasing longevity needs therefore to be wide-ranging. The present volume, while not aspiring to comprehensiveness or finality, endeavours to be a contribution to that debate. It is based upon presentations given at a conference at the Royal College of Physicians on the 4th December 1996. The range of invited speakers was intended, so far as possible within the compass of a one-day meeting, to reflect the breadth of the topic. The viewpoints of experts in biological gerontology, clinical medicine, demography, epidemiology, health economics and health care policy, sociology and medical ethics are represented. Ageing is a global issue and it is appropriate, therefore, that this book looks beyond the UK and indeed beyond developed countries, to developing countries where the rate of increase in the numbers of older people dwarfs that which is taking place in Europe and US.

It is inevitable that in the current politico-economic climate the issue of rationing, of prioritisation and competition for health care and other resources should be present explicitly and implicitly in several of the contributions. Their authors challenge the reader not only to address the issues but to think about them in a rather more sophisticated manner than is customary. The necessity of rationing is accepted; the acceptability of rationing according to age is not, nor is the inevitability of intergenerational conflict over access to care. Rationing of health and social care will be less Draconian if resources are used wisely. A critical evaluation of what is currently on offer – Is it effective? Is it efficient? – is essential, as is a recognition that early interventions may not only be desirable from the point of view of the patient but also be more cost-effective than postponing or denying definitive or adequate treatment. The demographic trends should not, in other words, feed assumptions about the need to limit the access of elderly people to appropriate medical care and social support, but should prompt hard thought about robust research into the ways in which the seeming necessity for rationing can be mitigated and irrational principles of rationing avoided.

The emphasis in this book is, inevitably, on health and social care. These are, of course, only means to an end and only part of a much bigger picture. One consequence of the demographic revolution should be a re-thinking of our sense of the course of life – and a recognition that, perhaps, after all, there is more to old age than loss and infirmity and the indignity of being reclassified as 'a burden' or 'a challenge'. Old age holds out promises as well as threats both for individuals and for society as a whole. Many are living to enjoy what Peter Laslett has christened the Third Age[5]: a period of health, often as long as childhood plus adolescence, free of the anxieties of child care and the pressures of work. Out of such elders, remote from the stereotypes of decrepitude, may come a new understanding of life: 'old men ought to be explorers'; old men and old women, students of the University of the Third Age, now can be.

In the conclusion to his Harveian Oration, which forms a fitting climax to this book, Professor Sir Grimley Evans urges that we should not let 'fears of what might be prevent our exploration of what could be'. He reflects that government is unlikely to provide the leadership and vision necessary to ensure that the implications of the demographic revolution are addressed.

The leadership will have to come from within the ranks of the knowledgeable and socially responsible citizenry.

It is hoped that *Increasing longevity: medical, social and political implications* will make a contribution to informing that 'knowledge-able and socially responsible citizenry'.

RAYMOND TALLIS
January 1998

References

1   Porter R. *The greatest benefit to mankind: A medical history of humanity from antiquity to the present.* London: Harper Collins, 1997.
2   *Idem, Ibid*, p178.
3   Manton KG, Corder L, Stallard E. Chronic disability trends in elderly United States populations: 1982-1994. *Proceedings of the National Academy of Sciences USA* 1997; **94**: 2593-8.
4   Fries JF, Crapo LM. *Vitality and Aging: Implications of the rectangular curve.* San Francisco: Freeman, 1981.
5   Laslett P. *A fresh map of life.* 2nd edn. London: Macmillan,1996.

Contents

1 | Population ageing over the next few decades

Anthony M Warnes
Professor of Social Gerontology, Centre for Ageing and Rehabilitation Studies, University of Sheffield

This chapter examines the recent and anticipated growth of the older population of Great Britain. It compares the British trends in longevity and age-specific death rates in later life with those of Europe. Switzerland has among the lowest mortality rates at the older ages in Europe, and the differentials for specific causes are examined. This information enables an assessment of this country's comparative successes and failures in combating mortality in later life and informs a discussion of the mortality assumptions in the current official population projections. The projection figures are reported, and the chapter concludes with comments on the importance to the health services of the expected number of older people, as opposed to their health status and treatment expectations.

Trends in life expectancy and age-specific death rates

'We are living longer' is a commonplace and true but inexact. While average life expectancy at birth has increased massively over the last century, the frequently presented figures misrepresent the practical change among people who survive infancy (Table 1). Overstatement arises because most of the improvement in survival has been in infant mortality, and the declines at later ages have been much less. Among males in England and Wales, the average annual increase in life expectancy at birth from the 1890s until 1990–92, was 0.7%, which compares with an annual rate of 0.2% for the mean remaining life expectancy at 65 years. There is also, however, an element of understatement because 'mean life expectancy' is calculated from a 'life table', a schedule of age-specific death rates in one or a few years. It is an unreal measure: the average survival of a newborn child that (impossibly) lives all

Table 1. The increase of life expectancy in England and Wales, 1891–1991

Base age	Mean life expectancy (years)				Annual rate of increase (%)			
	1891–1900	1950–52	1970–72	1990–92	1896–1991	1896–1951	1951–71	1971–91
Males								
E^0	44.1	66.4	69.0	73.2	0.53	0.73	0.19	0.30
E^{65}	10.3	11.7	12.2	14.2	0.34	1.23	0.21	0.76
E^{80}	4.2†	4.7	5.7*	6.4	0.44	0.20	0.88	0.65†
Females								
E^0	47.8	71.5	75.2	78.7	0.52	0.72	0.25	0.22
E^{65}	11.3	14.3	16.1	17.9	0.48	0.42	0.60	0.53
E^{80}	4.6†	5.0	7.3*	8.4	0.64	0.15	1.74	0.78†

E^x is the conventional notation for representing mean remaining expectancy of life at age x (in years) for a particular year or short period (indicated in the column headings)

* 1972–74; † 1973–91; ‡ Estimated from schedule of age-specific death rates

Source: OPCS (1994). *Mortality Statistics 1992: England and Wales, General*, HMSO, London, Table 15

its life in the short period covered by the life table. As the dominant mortality trend for a century has been reduction, period life expectancies have consistently underestimated the mean *actual* length of life. The recent acceleration of mortality declines at the older ages therefore raises considerable problems for forecasting methods and assumptions.[1]

The annual rate of improvement of remaining life expectancy at 65 years of age has risen during the second half of the present century and now is substantially greater than the improvement of life expectancy at birth (Table 1).[2] Among females, a strong acceleration at the oldest ages has recently occurred. These changes prompt the incorrect conclusion that improvements in survival during later life are now greater than in infancy. In fact, the annual reduction in infant mortality has recently been greater than before 1950 and remains much higher than the rate of decrease of death rates at 70 or 80 years of age (Table 2). The recent rate of late-age mortality declines is nonetheless striking. During the four successive 20-year periods from 1911–15 to 1991, the annual death rate at 85+ years in England and Wales decreased by 0.9, 7.8, 14.7 and 17.2% (the last figure for 1971–75 to 1991) (Table 2).

Recent trends in later life mortality in Britain and Europe by major causes

The publication in the United Nations Organisation's *Demographic yearbook* of late-age cause-specific death rates enables trends in Great Britain to be compared with those of other European countries.[3] Data are presented for eight broad groups of cause by sex, for five-year age groups of the older population (to 85+ years), and for 1960, 1970, 1980 and 1990. The figures are supplied by national statistics offices and are rigorously checked for reliability and validity. For some of the smaller countries, incomplete series are found and to maximise comparability they have been excluded. Full series for 20 nations have been used to compute population-weighted mean death rates for each condition, sex and year for the age groups 60–64, 70–74 and 80–84 years. The denominators are the estimated populations, also extracted from the *Demographic yearbooks* for the reference years.

Most attention is given to four dominant cause groups: cancers, cardiovascular disorders, cerebrovascular disorders and 'other' (including the still numerous deaths at the oldest ages from infectious and parasitic diseases, mainly of the respiratory and digestive systems). The remaining categories are diabetes,

Table 2. The acceleration of mortality improvement for both sexes in England and Wales, 1901–91

Age group (years)	Annual death rate per 1,000				Annual rate of decrease (%)			
	1901–05	1951–55	1971–75	1991	1903–91	1903–53	1953–73	1973–91
0–1	138	27	17	7	3.33	3.21	2.29	4.81
65–74	59.4	42.0	36.9	29.1	0.81	0.69	0.65	1.31
75–84	127.3	105.7	87.8	71.5	0.65	0.37	0.92	1.13

Percentage reduction in age-specific death rate during successive 20 years

Age group (years)	1911/5 to 1931/5	1931/5 to 1951/5	1951/5 to 1971/5	1971/5 to 1991
0–1	43.6	56.5	37.0	58.8
65–74	14.5	14.3	12.1	21.1
75–84	0.85	7.8	14.7	17.2

cirrhosis, accidents and undefined. A confounding factor is that since 1960 the attribution of causes of death has become more standardised across Europe (extensively discussed in UNO[3]). The 'undefined' share in 1960 was 1.7% for males and 1.9% for females, and by 1990 these percentages had declined to 0.3 and 0.4, respectively. It has been assumed that the causes of the 'undefined' deaths have the distribution of the reported causes.

In 1960 the male population-weighted all-cause death rate at age 60–64 years for the 20 European countries was 2,506 per 100,000 (or 2.5%) and the female rate was 1,327 (1.3%) (Table 3). The male rate decreased by one-fifth during 1960–90 and the female rate by nearly one-third. In 1960, the male 70–74 years death rate was 2.4 times higher than at 60–64 years, and that at 80–84 years was six times higher. The age differentials among females were greater. Over the three decades, male death rates decreased by around 0.75% per year in all three age groups, while the female death rates decreased more but with greater variation by age.

The trends for each age group and each sex vary intricately but Figs 1 and 2 display the main features. Beginning with the share of deaths from cardiovascular causes, this increased during the 1960s and 1970s, particularly at the younger ages, but during the 1980s fell sharply. The share of deaths from cerebrovascular causes declined consistently through the three decades, while that from cancers has increased throughout. By 1990, cancers were the dominant cause at 60–64 years, but among males aged 80–84 years their frequency was just one-third of the cardiovascular and cerebrovascular causes. Another striking feature is the continuing large share for the 'other' causes. These account for more than 20% of deaths in all three age groups of men and women, with the highest shares at the oldest ages and among males.

The UK male rates improved relative to Europe whereas the female rates worsened, particularly at 60–64 and 70–74 years. For UK males aged 60–64 years, the 11% 'excess' of deaths in 1960 declined to a 6% 'deficit' in 1990 (Table 4). At 70–74 years, the 12% 'excess' of deaths in 1960 halved by 1990, and there was a small relative improvement at 80–84 years. For UK females aged 60–64 years, the excess of deaths increased from 4% in 1960 to 23% in 1990; for those aged 70–74 years, a small deficit became an excess of 11%; and for those aged 80–84 years, the 7% deficit in 1960 hardly changed.

The period saw a serious deterioration of mortality among men in eastern Europe.[4] Without this, the UK trends would have been less favourable as shown by comparisons with Switzerland (Table 4,

Table 3. Trends in late age mortality in 20 European countries, 1960–90

Age group	Death rate per 100,000				Annual change (%)			
	1960	1970	1980	1990	1960–70	1970–80	1980–90	1960–90
Males								
60–64	2,506	2,465	2,185	2,008	−0.17	−1.20	−0.84	−0.74
70–74	5,926	6,181	5,556	4,712	+0.42	−1.06	−1.63	−0.76
80–84	15,114	14,081	13,475	12,025	−0.71	−0.44	−1.13	−0.76
Females								
60–64	1,327	1,205	1,029	907	−0.96	−1.57	−1.25	−1.26
70–74	4,017	3,646	2,989	2,510	−0.96	−1.97	−1.73	−1.56
80–84	12,317	10,911	9,588	8,067	−1.21	−1.28	−1.71	−1.40

The 20 nations are Austria, Belgium, Bulgaria, Czechoslovakia, Denmark, Finland, France, Germany (FDR), Greece, Hungary, Ireland, Italy, Netherlands, Norway, Poland, Portugal, Spain, Sweden, Switzerland and the United Kingdom

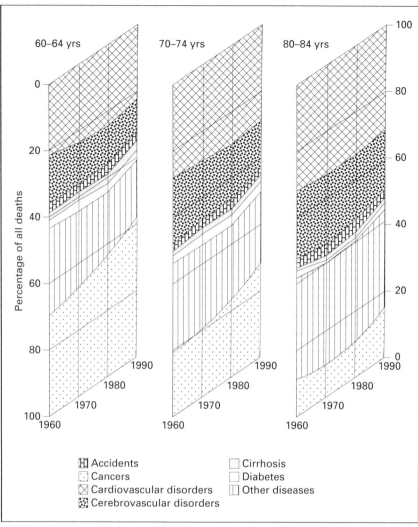

Fig 1. *The changing distribution of male deaths by cause at ages 60–64, 70–74 and 80–84 years: population-weighted mean death rates for 20 European countries, 1960, 1970, 1980 and 1990.* (The 20 included countries are: Austria, Belgium, Bulgaria, Czechoslovakia, Denmark, Finland, France, Germany (FDR), Greece, Hungary, Ireland, Italy, Netherlands, Norway, Poland, Portugal, Spain, Sweden, Switzerland and the UK. For sources of data see text and reference 3.)

C columns). In 1960 the UK rates were higher than the Swiss for all male age groups and the differentials had increased by 1990. The relative deterioration was, however, much greater for the two younger female age groups: among those aged 60–64 years, a 7% excess of deaths in 1960 increased to 64% by 1990.

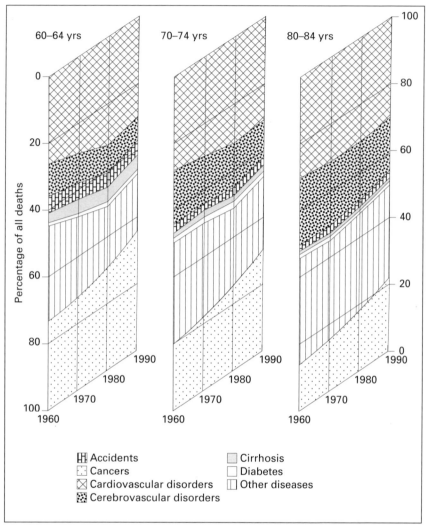

Fig 2. *The changing distribution of female deaths by cause at ages 60–64, 70–74 and 80–84 years: population-weighted mean death rates for 20 European countries, 1960, 1970, 1980 and 1990*

The cause-specific comparisons show that Switzerland generally achieved much greater overall reductions in cancer, cardiovascular, stroke and 'other' deaths than the UK, particularly at the younger elderly ages and among females (Table 5). Among these four causes, the only instances of the UK improvement exceeding the Swiss were in cancer and 'other' deaths among males aged 60–64 years, and in cardiovascular deaths among males aged 80–84 years. The markedly worse death rates in 1990 among young elderly

Table 4. Trends in late age mortality in the UK relative to both Europe and Switzerland, 1960–90

Age group	A. Death rate per 100,000			B. UK/E^{20}* rates				C. UK/Swiss rates			
	1960	1980	1990	1960	1970	1980	1990	1960	1970	1980	1990
Males											
60–64	2,788	2,363	1,894	1.11	1.10	1.08	0.94	1.18	1.28	1.29	1.24
70–74	6,642	6,054	4,976	1.12	1.11	1.09	1.06	1.18	1.24	1.27	1.27
80–84	15,524	14,309	12,047	1.03	1.07	1.06	1.00	1.05	1.11	1.17	1.12
Females											
60–64	1,380	1,236	1,116	1.04	1.08	1.20	1.23	1.07	1.28	1.49	1.64
70–74	3,908	3,160	2,797	0.97	1.00	1.06	1.11	1.01	1.12	1.31	1.45
80–84	11,459	9,101	7,696	0.93	0.94	0.95	0.95	0.92	0.95	1.13	1.15

* E20 refers to the population-weighted mean rate for 20 European countries listed in Table 3

Table 5. Ratios of UK to Swiss cause-specific death rates, 60–64 and 80–84 years by sex, 1960 and 1990

Causes of death	Males						Females					
	60–64 years			80–84 years			60–64 years			80–84 years		
	1960	1990	* %	1960	1990	* %	1960	1990	* %	1960	1990	* %
Cancers	1.18	1.14	-3.2	0.87	1.00	14.1	1.02	1.40	37.8	0.78	1.05	33.7
Cardiovascular	1.42	**1.71**	20.6	1.08	1.04	-3.5	1.19	**2.62**	120.7	0.87	1.07	23.3
Cerebrovascular	1.46	**1.79**	22.4	1.13	1.39	23.1	**1.81**	**2.84**	56.6	1.14	**1.57**	37.3
Other	1.29	1.22	-5.1	1.12	**1.51**	34.5	0.89	**1.91**	113.8	0.94	1.40	49.0
Diabetes	0.37	0.94	155.1	0.82	0.84	2.9	0.48	0.99	105.9	0.51	0.54	6.1
Cirrhosis	0.12	0.45	265.6	0.15	0.28	83.2	0.63	0.83	31.6	0.30	0.70	130.8
Accidents	0.46	0.46	0.2	0.68	0.31	-54.0	1.00	0.64	-36.0	0.77	0.35	-54.4
All causes	1.18	1.24	5.8	1.05	1.12	6.8	1.07	**1.64**	53.4	0.92	1.15	24.6

UK : Swiss ratios in excess of 1.5 are in bold type
* % is the percentage change of the UK : Swiss ratio during 1960–90

females stand out in the table. Over the three decades, the worst comparative deterioration was in cirrhosis deaths among young elderly males, although the UK rate in 1990 was still less than half the Swiss rate, but among the four most prevalent causes, the sharp relative increase in female cardiovascular mortality at 60–64 years will be of greatest concern to both health promotion and clinical professionals. Cancer death rates for UK males kept close to the Swiss trends and the 1960 excess of deaths was slightly reduced among those aged 60–64 years.

In 1990 countries as diverse as Switzerland, France, Spain, Norway, Sweden, the Netherlands and Austria had lower mortality rates among older people than Great Britain.[5,6] Although some part of our disadvantage may stem from harsher living conditions at birth, in childhood and during the working years of today's older population, other influential factors include current lifestyles, nutrition and medical care. The lowest mortality rates in Europe are feasible targets for this country. Many reactions to the prospective ageing of our population negatively focus on rising care demands and the financial implications. A positive approach, to identify and pursue the ways in which the health and survival of the older population can be improved, would be a welcome corrective.

Population projections

Through this century, the total number of births in England and Wales has ranged from under 6.5 million during the 1930s and 1970s to 9.3 million during the first decade and over 8 million during the 1910s and 1960s (Table 6). While survival has improved and net migration change has altered, the decade-by-decade fluctuation in the population 'at risk' of reaching old age not only indicates likely changes in the size of the older population but reminds us that the older population, like that of school age, rises and falls.

The absolute and relative size of the future elderly population cannot be known precisely. Population projections are a function of the assumptions about fertility, mortality and sometimes migration built into them, and are therefore as good as our understanding and models of recent trends. That understanding has been improving fast but remains imperfect. Demographers have tended to see all-age mortality as steadily declining, but have difficulties in setting the assumptions for late-age mortality. To the growing awareness of the gentle acceleration of late age mortality decline

Table 6. Live births in England and Wales, 1911–90

Birth decade	Births (thousands)	Change on prior decade (%)	Attains age 60+	Attains age 80+
1911–20	8,096	−10.8	1970s	1990s
1921–30	7,127	−12.0	1980s	2000s
1931–40	6,065	−14.9	1990s	2010s
1941–50	7,251	+19.6	2000s	2020s
1951–60	7,075	−2.4	2010s	2030s
1961–70	8,326	+17.7	2020s	2040s
1971–80	6,472	−22.3	2030s	2050s
1981–90	6,613	+2.2	2040s	2060s

Sources: OPCS (1987) *Birth statistics: historical series of statistics from registrations of births in England and Wales, 1837–1983.* OPCS (1991) *Population Trends,* **66,** Table 9

has recently been added evidence of increases in male death rates in early adulthood:

> For men between the ages of 24 and 46 mortality rates are tending to rise at present, largely due to deaths arising from HIV infection, but also from an increasing number of suicides and accidental deaths. ... Past and current trends suggest that those now over about age 47 will continue to show, in each cohort, lower mortality rates than in the preceding cohort ... this has been their experience to date and at present their mortality rates are diminishing by between one and four per cent a year. This trend has been strong for nearly two decades. ... It has therefore been decided to assume, in general, rather greater improvement than in the previous projections for all those born in 1945 or earlier.[7]

A selection of the official projections is given in Table 7. These suggest that the UK population aged 60+ years will exceed 12 million during the 1990s and in the early decades of the next century enter a period of faster growth, to 15.8 million by 2021. During the 2030s the growth phase will end and it is expected that during 2041–2061 the 60+ years population will fall by 6% to 17.1 million (reflecting the low birth rates of the 1970s). During this period the total population is likely to be falling and the share in the older age groups will be sustained but will not grow substantially. In 2031 those aged 60+ years are likely to form 29.1% of the total, and over the following thirty years the projections suggest that the share will increase by just 0.7%. An increasing average age is projected among

Table 7. Projected number of elderly people by age: UK, 2001–2061

Year	Population (millions)				Share of total (%)			Annual growth (%) *		
	60+	70+	80+	All ages	60+	70+	80+	60+	70+	80+
2001	12.2	6.8	2.5	59.7	20.4	11.4	4.2	0.2	0.8	1.6
2011	13.9	7.1	2.9	61.1	22.8	11.7	4.7	1.3	0.5	1.3
2021	15.8	8.7	3.2	62.0	25.4	14.1	5.2	1.2	2.0	1.2
2031	18.1	10.0	4.3	62.1	29.1	16.1	6.9	1.4	1.4	3.0
2041	17.9	11.4	4.8	61.0	29.3	18.6	7.9	-0.1	1.3	1.2
2051	17.5	10.6	5.4	59.3	29.4	18.0	9.1	-0.2	-0.7	1.1
2061	17.1	10.3	4.7	57.4	29.8	17.9	8.2	-0.2	-0.4	-1.3

*Average annual growth rate over previous decade, calculated from full figures
Source: OPCS (1993) *National population projections 1991–2061*. Appendix 1, pp 32–3

the elderly population, and the numbers aged over 75 years will grow more quickly than the entire elderly population.

During the 2020s, the 1960s high birth cohorts will enter their seventh decade of life. Consequently the decade will see an exceptionally large increase (projected to be 14.9%) of the 60–69 years population. Rarely emphasised, however, is that during the following decade the low 1970s birth cohort will reach their seventh decade and so the population aged 60–69 years is projected to fall, not by a small margin but by 1.57 million or 19.4%. During the 2030s and subsequent decades, there may as a result be difficult issues of retrenchment in some health services for elderly people. Thirty-five years is a long way ahead but, whether witting or unconscious, there is a touch of deception in spotlighting projections for the 2020s without mentioning the prospects beyond. The target date 2030 maximises the prospective rate of increase and is therefore most useful to those keen to demonstrate a 'tidal wave'.

Conclusion: how important are the projected numbers?

In considering the impact on Britain's health services of improvements in longevity and of population ageing, the projected numbers are but a starting point.[8,9] Demographers and epidemiologists go one step further and seek reliable time series of the dependency and health status of the population. The latest evidence from the United States is building a substantial case that age-specific disability levels in that country are falling.[10,11] Increasingly it is realised that the relationships between population size and the demand for health services are more complex.[12] Recent years have seen substantial rises in health service consultation and contact rates in most developed nations. Utilisation is booming, and from all age groups. There is little understanding and, remarkably, there are hardly any formal models of the factors that influence patients' presentation. Whether from increased numbers, or from rising demands, the health and elderly care complexes are likely for many decades to witness increasing demands for their services. Rising longevity has only a small part in this. The training and financial implications are clear, but only Treasury ministers should see the anticipated growth as largely problematic. A greater danger within the health services is that the accommodation of growth will conspire with evidence of some absolute improvements in elderly people's health and survival to instil complacency. In comparison to many comparable countries in Europe, the health and survival of Britain's elderly people is slipping. It is important to understand the reasons for this, and to attempt to reverse the trend.

References

1   Murphy M. The prospect of mortality: England and Wales and the United States of America, 1962–89. *British Actuarians Journal* 1995; **1**: 330–50.

2   Grundy E. The epidemiology of aging. In: Brocklehurst JC, Tallis R, Fillit H (eds). *Textbook of geriatric medicine and gerontology.* Edinburgh: Churchill Livingstone, 1992.

3   United Nations Organisation. *Demographic yearbook 1993: Special Issue, Population aging and the situation of elderly persons.* New York: UNO, 1993.

4   United Nations Organisation. The demography of countries with economies in transition. In *World population prospects: The 1994 revision.* New York: Population Division, Department of Economic and Social Information and Policy Analysis, UNO, 1995: 21–39.

5   Caselli G. *Long-term trends in European mortality.* London: Office of Population Censuses and Surveys, 1994. (Studies on Medical and Population Subjects No. 56).

6   Warnes AM. Demographic ageing in Europe: trends and policy responses. In: Noin D, Woods RI (eds). *The changing population of Europe.* Oxford: Blackwell, 1993: 82–99.

7   Office of Population Censuses and Surveys. *National population projections: 1991-based* (Series PP2, No. 18). London: HMSO, 1993: 8.

8   Central Health Monitoring Unit. *The health of elderly people: An epidemiological overview,* Volume 1 and Companion Papers. London: HMSO, 1992.

9   Medical Research Council. *The health of the UK's elderly people: Topic review.* London: MRC, 1994.

10 Crimmins EM, Saito Y, Reynolds SL. Further evidence on recent trends in the prevalence and incidence of disability among older Americans from two sources: the LSOA and NHIS. *Journal of Gerontology: Social Sciences* 1997; **52B**(2): S59–S71.

11 Manton KG, Corder L, Stallard E. Chronic disability trends in elderly United States populations: 1982–1994. *Proceedings of the National Academy of Sciences* 1997; **94**(6): 2593–8.

12 Charlton J, Murphy M (eds). *The health of adult Britain 1841–1994,* Office for National Statistics, Decennial Supplement 12. London: HMSO, 1997.

2 | Ageing, ill health and disability

Emily Grundy
Reader in Social Gerontology, Centre for Population Studies,
London School of Hygiene and Tropical Medicine

Relationships between ageing, ill health and disability are, given the demographic context outlined in Chapter 1, clearly of crucial importance in contemporary developed societies. Unfortunately our knowledge of these relationships is still patchy and we do not yet know enough to answer definitively some very important questions about whether people are getting healthier or less healthy at particular ages.[1]

Changes in survival to later life

One issue about which there can be no question is the marked improvement in the proportion of successive 20th century birth cohorts who have survived to older ages. Figure 1 shows the survivorship of men and women born in 1905 in England and Wales compared with that of later born cohorts. As can be seen there has been a very considerable improvement in the prospects of surviving to maturity. Reductions in mortality have been greatest in younger age groups and the curves show a trend towards 'rectangularisation'. However, there have also been changes at the oldest end of the distribution. Analyses of data from Japan, the US and Sweden show a recent slight widening of the distribution of ages of death,[2] contrary to the continuing compression of mortality hypothesised by Fries.[3]

One result of these changes in survival coupled with the change in the age structure of the population, which is mainly due to long-term declines in fertility rates, is that the majority of deaths now occur in elderly people. As shown in Table 1, well over half of all deaths are now among people over 75 and only 1% among 0–4-year-olds. This is important because many of the health care demands and health care costs attributed to ageing populations are really to do with death and dying; if age at death is postponed

17

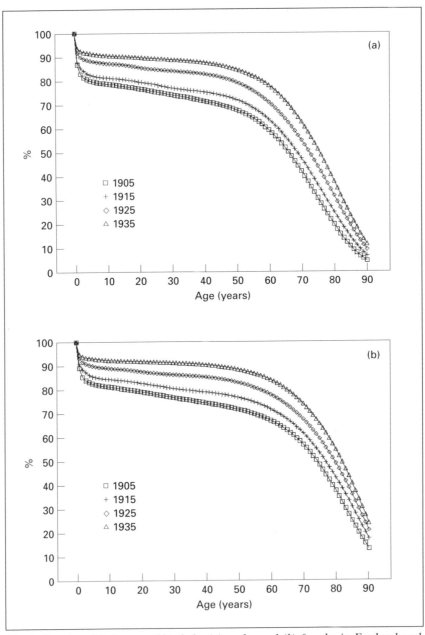

Fig 1. *Survivorship by year of birth for (a) males and (b) females in England and Wales.* Source: Grundy[1]

to later life, which I am sure everyone would see as a desirable outcome, then some health care needs will also be shifted to later life.

Table 1. Deaths at ages 0–4 and 75+, England and Wales, 1901 and 1994

| | % of all deaths at ages: | |
Year	0–4	75+
1901	37	12
1994	1	58

Sources: UN and OPCS reported in Grundy 1997[13]

Age at which 15 years of life remains

One way of examining changes in mortality and survival is to consider trends in the age at which on average further life expectancy equals 15 years, as shown in Fig 2. In the post-World War II period, the age at which this 'threshold' is reached has increased quite considerably, particularly since the 1960s, and now stands at 68 for women and 62 for men, compared with 61–62 for women and 57–58 for men in 1951.[4] It has been argued by some[5] that this is the kind of information we should use to define later life and that perhaps eligibility for pensions and so forth should be related to these types of data, rather than fixed at an age decided upon fifty years ago.

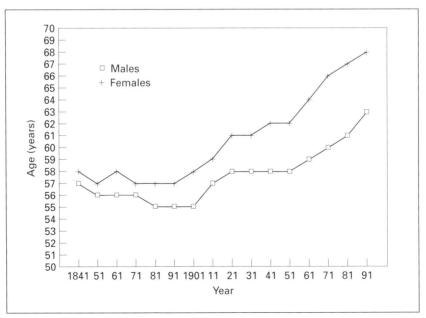

Fig 2. *Age at which 15 years of life remain by period and sex.* Source: Grundy[4]

The health status of the elderly population

What are the implications of these changes in mortality for the health status of the elderly population? Broadly speaking there are two main camps of opinion. One rather pessimistic one suggests that as more people survive to later life, those with unfavourable health legacies comprise a larger proportion of the total. This, it has been argued, coupled with medical interventions that may prolong the period of pre-death morbidity, results in older populations becoming less healthy.[6,7] More optimistic commentators argue that later cohorts have a better health legacy reflecting better child nutrition, less exposure to infection and more education, and so should have better health throughout their lives. Recent improvements in mortality, it is argued, reflect these gains and success in postponing, if not preventing altogether, the onset of degenerative diseases. Better management of degenerative diseases, it is suggested, may also have resulted in postponement of the onset of disability.[3,8]

One of the problems in trying to resolve this important debate is the difficulty involved in measuring health at the population level. A range of measures, including data on mortality, morbidity and disability, are used to address this issue. There is also growing support for the use of measures of mortality and morbidity and disability in combination to produce estimates of 'healthy' or 'disability-free' life expectancy.

In this country and the United States activities of daily living scales (ADLs) are frequently used as a measure of functional disability, although the World Health Organization (WHO) is now promoting the use of approaches based on the *International classification of impairment, disabilities and handicaps.*[9] Survey data on self-reported health and even broader concepts such as well-being are also advocated by some on the grounds that we should not just look at whether people have particular conditions, but more broadly at how they feel about their health.

Cross-sectional data on ageing, health and disability

Prevalence rates of all indicators of health show strong relationships with age. Cross-sectional data on long-term illness from the 1991 population census are shown in Fig 3 for those living in private (ordinary) households and those in institutions (non-private households). There is a steady increase in the prevalence of this indicator of poor health until the mid-50s or so, then a sharper

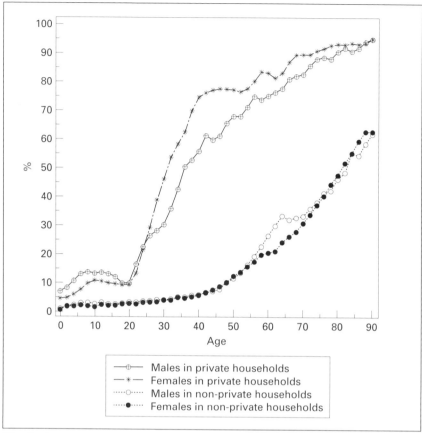

Fig 3. *Limiting long-term illness: sex and residential status, GB 1991 (non-private household data have been smoothed).* Source: Census Sample of Anonymised Records data reported in Glaser, Murphy and Grundy[14]

rise, particularly in oldest age groups. Similarly, indicators of use of health services, such as inpatient stays, also show a strong relationship with age (Fig 4). These data on hospital activity differ slightly from data on use of community services, in that use of hospital services in elderly age groups tends to be higher among men, whereas use of domiciliary services such as home helps or district nurses is higher among women.[1] This is partly because more women live alone and so have less help available from co-residents; it also reflects differences by gender in the timing and cause distribution of death.

Data from the Health Survey for England, and all other similar sources, show a very high prevalence of musculoskeletal disorders, among women in particular, and of heart and circulatory system disorders, particularly among men (Table 2). Over a third of

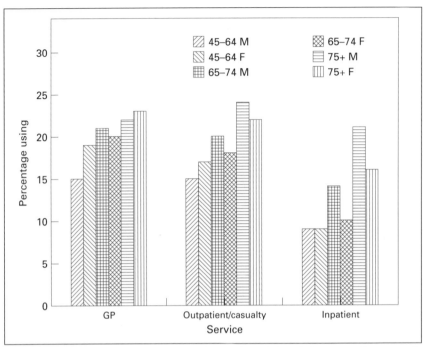

Fig 4. *Percentage consulting an NHS GP in the 14 days before interview; attending an outpatient/casualty department in the preceding three months; or with an inpatient stay in the last year, Britain 1994.* Source: OPCS[15]

women and a quarter of men over the age of 65 report a musculoskeletal disorder; a third of men and a quarter of women report a disorder of the heart and circulatory system.

In terms of effect of health problems on activities, data from the 1994 General Household Survey again show quite strong relationships with age, particularly in measures which are based on people's abilities to undertake various activities. So, for example, about a half of women over 85 report being unable to manage one or more locomotion activities, such as getting up and down stairs, getting around the house, or getting outside the house on their own. These prevalence rates, especially in the oldest age groups, are *under-estimates* because this survey does not include the population in institutions, who have much higher rates of disability (Fig 3) and comprise a large proportion of the seriously disabled. Responses to more general questions on health, such as whether respondents had a long-standing illness which limited their activities or how respondents rated their health, were less strongly associated with age, but show a high prevalence of health problems in elderly age groups. Responses to these types of question are

Table 2. Rate per 1,000 of long-standing illness or disability by condition group, England 1993, private household population aged 65+

Condition group (ICD chapter, 9th revision)	Men Prevalence	Rank	Women Prevalence	Rank
Musculoskeletal system	264	2	388	1
Heart and circulatory system	342	1	262	2
Respiratory system	135	3	92	4
Digestive system	86	4	94	3
Endocrine and metabolic	75	5	79	5
Eye complaints	56	6	63	6

ICD: International Classification of Diseases (WHO)
Source: OPCS[16]

known to be very strongly influenced by health expectations and what people think is appropriate for their age.

The high prevalence rates of specific and more general health problems and conditions shown in Tables 2 and 3 present a rather depressing view of the relationship between ageing, health and disability. However, it is important to remember that for many people who report having a musculoskeletal disorder or a

Table 3. Indicators of health problems/disability by age and sex, Great Britain 1994 (private household population only)

Percentage reporting		65–69	70–74	Age 75–79	80–84	85+	65+
Limiting	M	39	38	42	50	43	40
long-standing illness	F	35	41	43	46	54	42
Inability to	M	8	7	9	21	22	10
manage one or more locomotion activities on own	F	10	13	19	27	50	19
Inability to	M	3	5	6	12	17	6
usually manage bathing/showering/ washing all over on own	F	5	7	9	15	23	10
Health in general in	M	21	20	22	31	17	22
preceding year 'not good'	F	18	24	27	26	30	24

Source: OPCS[15]

circulatory disorder or some other condition, the effects on their
health status and ability to carry out normal activities may not
always be very serious. Figure 5, based on data from the General
Household Survey, shows that only about 40% of women over 75
with musculoskeletal disorders consider that their health is poor.
Women with respiratory diseases, the overall prevalence of which is
lower, include a higher proportion who feel that their health is not
good. This raises an interesting question about how to assess the
burden of a particular disease as such an approach needs to take
account of both the prevalence (the proportions affected) and the
consequences of having the condition.

Trends in health: examples from US data on heart disease

The results shown above are cross-sectional ones from one point in
time. In terms of trying to understand the relationship between
ageing, ill health and disability they may be distorted because of
strong cohort differences in health patterns. Clearly they also cannot reveal anything about trends over time. Below we consider
various trend data relevant to the hypotheses about possible

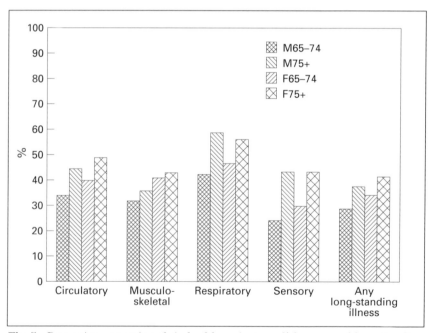

Fig 5. *Proportions reporting their health as 'not good' by cause of long-standing
illness.* Source: analysis of General Household Survey data reported in
Grundy[4]

changes in the health of the older population taking as an example trends in heart disease in the United States.

Table 4 shows the prevalence of self-reported ischaemic heart disease in 1979–81 and 1985–87. There appear to have been huge increases between the late 1970s and mid to late 1980s in the proportion of people reporting this type of heart disease. During the same period, as shown in Table 5, there were big falls in death rates from diseases of the heart. These tables can be interpreted in various ways. One possibility is that the incidence of heart disease has remained the same but that people are surviving longer with

Table 4. Percentage of population reporting ischaemic heart disease, US 1979–81 to 1985–87

Age and sex	Period 1979–81	1985–87	Percentage change
Males			
55–64	7.8	9.9	+26.9
65–74	13.4	15.1	+11.3
75+	10.7	15.6	+14.6
Females			
55–64	4.2	4.5	+10.7
65–74	8.3	8.5	+10.2
75+	9.8	12.0	+12.2

Source: National Health Interview Survey data reported by Mermelstein *et al*[17]

Table 5. Percentage change in death rates for diseases of the heart, US 1980–86

Age	Male	Female
55–59	−18.9	−13.8
60–64	−16.5	−10.7
65–69	−18.2	−13.3
70–74	−14.9	−12.7
75–79	−13.0	−12.8
80–84	−10.3	−11.4
85+	− 9.6	− 6.3

Source: National Health Interview Survey data reported in Furner, Maurer and Rosenberg[18]

the condition, and with associated disabilities, leading to higher prevalence rates. This would suggest a deterioration in health of the population.

A second interpretation might be that incidence rates had remained unchanged and survival with the disease increased, but that this reflects successes in postponing the more serious consequences of the condition, including both disability and death. This would mean an increase in prevalence of the condition, but not necessarily any increase in the prevalence of more serious disabilities associated with it.

A third possible explanation is that the increased self-reporting of ischaemic heart disease reflects a change in health expectations and health awareness, rather than any 'real' change in prevalence. There is some evidence to support this third hypothesis. Data from the United States on hypertension (Table 6) show very substantial differences between self-reported hypertension and prevalence rates derived from blood pressure measurements taken by nurses. Prevalence rates based on measurements taken by nurses show little change between the early 1970s and late 1970s, whereas prevalence rates based on self-reports show substantial increases. This suggests an increase in health awareness (which might be interpreted as a positive indicator) rather than an increase in the prevalence of the condition.

Healthy life expectancy

As discussed earlier, an increasingly common approach to the measurement of health in later life is to combine data on morbidity with mortality data to partition life expectancy into 'healthy' and 'unhealthy' components. Of course the results of such calculations reflect the quality of the inputs. If the trend data on morbidity are influenced by changes in health expectations or otherwise biased, then the estimates of health expectancy will also be flawed. However, some results from large longitudinal studies including detailed health measurements are available. Manton and Stallard[8] report findings from the National Long-Term Care Survey in the United States, a prospective study of elderly people with some initial disability which includes the institutional and the general population. These results indicate a significant improvement between the early and late 1980s in the proportion of further life expectancy at age 85 that was classified as active or disability free; from 62% to 73%. Manton and Stallard attribute this partly to improvements in the educational status of the population. In both

Table 6. Hypertension in the US

Measured by nurse
NHANES
Definite hypertension (≥160/95)

| | % | |
	1971–4	1976–80
Males – white		
55–64	38	38
65–74	41	44
Males – black		
55–64	54	54
65–74	59	45
Females – white		
55–64	39	39
65–74	53	53
Females – black		
55–64	64	62
65–74	69	77

Self-reported
NHIS
Reported hypertension

| | % | |
	1972	1979–81
Males		
55–64	14.8	27.5
65–74	18.2	30.6
Females		
55–64	21.9	29.6
65–74	30.4	41.2

NHANES: National Health and Nutrition Examination Survey; NHIS: National
Health Interview Survey
Source: NHIS and NHANES data reported in Grundy[17]

periods those with more that nine years of education had a higher
ratio of active to disabled life expectancy than those with less
education, but improvements between the two periods were
greatest for those with less education.

As yet we lack comparable longitudinal data from Britain. However, some estimates from cross-sectional data in the General Household Survey suggest a recent reduction in the extent of serious disability in the very old population. For example in 1991, 79% of men and 80% of women over 85 could bathe themselves, feed themselves, get in and out of bed, and get to the toilet without help compared with only 69% and 64% of men and women of this age in 1980.[1] This survey excludes those in institutions and the size of this excluded group increased during the 1980s; however, estimates allowing for this factor also show an improvement.[10] During the same period, however, self-reported long-term illness tends to have increased, possibly reflecting changes in health expectations and/or some increase in the extent of less serious disability. This is in line with trends reported for other European countries.[11] One interpretation of these trends is that they may be due to successful secondary and tertiary preventive interventions postponing or preventing the progression from morbidity to serious disability.

The future

Finally, I want to have a look into the future and consider the implications of further mortality decline for the age composition of the population. A team at the United Nations[12] has derived estimates of what they term 'limit' mortality, that is very low mortality levels assuming substantial falls in major causes of death. This level of mortality would result in a life expectancy at birth of 91, some 17 years longer than the present level. Applying these mortality rates, and constant fertility rates, to the population of Western Europe as composed in the late 1980s would result in a population in which a third were aged 60 and over and 14% aged 75 and over by the period 2020–2025.[12] Given the strong associations between age and rates of long-term illness and disability considered here, such a change would imply an enormous increase in the need for health and support services. However, if the threshold of morbidity and disability can be pushed back, just as the age at which 15 years of life remains has changed (and would change further under these mortality assumptions) then the outcome of such a demographic scenario would not be the disaster it might appear. This implies a need for great efforts in research and practice and also a change in attitudes, so that 75-year-olds in the future do not have the same health and activity profiles of 75-year-olds today.

References

1 Grundy E. Population Review: (5) The population aged 60 and over. *Population Trends* 1996; **84**: 14–20.

2 Wilmoth JR, Curtsinger JW, Horiuchi S. Rectangularization revisited; survival curves for humans and fruit flies. Annual Meeting of the Population Association of America, San Francisco, 1995.

3 Fries JF. Aging, natural death, and the compression of morbidity. *New England Journal of Medicine* 1980; **303**: 130–5.

4 Grundy E. The health of older adults 1841–1991. In: Charlton JC, Murphy M (eds). *The health of adult Britain.* London: HMSO, 1997.

5 Siegel JS. *A generation of change: A profile of America's older population.* New York: Russell Sage Foundation, 1993.

6 Gruenberg EM. The failure of success. *Millbank Memorial Fund Quarterly* 1977; **55**: 3–24.

7 Verbrugge L. Longer life but worsening health: trends in health and mortality in middle-aged and older persons. *Millbank Memorial Fund Quarterly* 1984; **62**: 475–519.

8 Manton K, Stallard E. Medical demography: interaction of disability dynamics and mortality. In: Martin LG, Preston SH (eds). *Demography of aging.* Washington DC: National Academy Press, 1994.

9 World Health Organization. *International classification of impairments, disabilities and handicaps.* Geneva: WHO, 1980.

10 Bone MR, Bebbington AC, Jagger C, Morgan K, Nicolaas G. *Health expectancy and its uses.* London: HMSO, 1995.

11 Boshuizen HC, van de Water HPA. *An international comparison of health expectancies.* Leiden: TNO Health Research, 1994.

12 Gonnot J-P. Some selected aspects of mortality in the ECE region. In: *United Nations Economic Commission for Europe, Demographic causes and economic consequences of population aging.* New York: United Nations, 1992.

13 Grundy EMD. Population dynamics and health. In: Detels R, Holland W, McEwen J, Ommen G (eds). *Oxford textbook of public health*, 3rd edn, Vol 1. Oxford: Oxford University Press, 1997: 75–94.

14 Glaser K, Murphy M, Grundy E. Limiting long-term illness and household structure among people aged 45 and over, Great Britain 1991. *Ageing and Society* 1997; **17**: 3–19.

15 Office of Population Censuses and Surveys. *Living in Britain, report on the General Household Survey 1994.* London: HMSO.

16 Office of Population Censuses and Surveys. *Health survey for England 1993.* London: HMSO, 1995.

17 Mermelstein R, Miller B, Prohanska T, Benson V, Van Nostrand JF. Measures of health. In: Van Nostrand JF, Furner DE, Suzman R (eds). *Health data on older Americans: United States 1992.* National Center for Health Statistics, Vital Health Statistics (27). Hyattsville, Maryland: US Department of Health and Human Services, 1993.

18 Furner SE, Maurer J, Rosenberg H. Mortality. In: Van Nostrand JF, Furner DE, Suzman, R (eds). *Health data on older Americans: United States 1992.* National Center for Health Statistics, Vital Health Statistics (27). Hyattsville, Maryland: US Department of Health and Human Services, 1993.

19 Grundy EMD. The epidemiology of aging. In: Brocklehurst JC, Tallis R, Fillit H (eds). *Textbook of geriatric medicine and gerontology*, 4th edn. Edinburgh: Churchill Livingstone, 1992: 3–20.

3 | Increasing longevity: the economic implications

Alan Maynard

Professor of Health Economics, York Health Economics Consortium, University of York

Economics is the science of choice. Resources always and everywhere are scarce and everyone, be they individuals, groups or societies, have to choose how to allocate these scarce resources amongst competing activities. In health care, as in every other activity, this involves decision-makers choosing to do one thing and to give up another. The value of the forgone alternative is the opportunity cost.

All choices have opportunity costs. A decision to give an 85-year-old man a coronary heart bypass means that funds are used which could otherwise have been used to treat a middle-aged woman with multiple sclerosis with the drug interferon beta. The decision not to treat Child B freed tens of thousands of pounds worth of resources which could fund hip replacements for the elderly or many other interventions for the population.

The impact of increasing longevity, with or without the morbidity characteristics of existing cohorts of the elderly, will, because of technological change and public expectations, make choices about who will live in what degree of pain and discomfort, and who, in extremis, will be left to die, even more difficult. Such choices should be made in relation to explicit criteria and determined by society in an open fashion so that we not only know our fates but also that those who determine our fates, whether clinician, politician, manager or family, are accountable. But what criteria should be used to determine who gets access to what health care in the UK National Health Service?

Rationing by the effectiveness criterion

Recently there has been much advocacy of 'evidence-based medicine' (EBM). One school of EBM advocates is led by Professor David Sackett of the UK Cochrane Centre in Oxford. He and his colleagues have argued:[1]

Doctors practising evidence based medicine will identify and apply
the most efficacious interventions to maximise the quality and
quantity of life for individual patients. This may raise rather than
lower the costs of their care.

Apart from the paternalism in the phrase 'will identify and apply',
implying no patient choice and which the authors have now con-
ceded as inappropriate, there are other problems associated with
this 'efficacy' approach. The judgement of efficacy has to be made
from the systematic review of well designed randomised control
trials (RCTs). Typically the patient entry criteria to such trials are
very strict, often with elderly people being excluded. Moreover, the
administration of the new treatment (eg a new drug) is carefully
supervised to ensure compliance, which may not reflect 'real world'
practice once the intervention is in general use. As a consequence,
interventions may prove efficacious in trials but may not always be
so when in general use because of inappropriate treatment decisions
by doctors and poor maintenance practices by patients.

However, let us assume that a treatment (B) is proved to be
efficacious and effective and the characteristics of it and the
alternative (A) are:

- Treatment A: produces 7 quality adjusted life years (or QALYs).
- Treatment B: produces 15 quality adjusted life years (or QALYs).

If effectiveness is the rationing criterion, clinicians would opt for
treatment B. However, such a choice ignores cost and the fact that
budgets are limited.

Rationing by the efficiency criterion

Decision-makers in the UK NHS are required to allocate resources
to competing patients not on the basis of their willingness and
ability to pay (as in private markets) but in relation to 'need'. If
need is defined as the patient's capacity to benefit from care per
unit of cost, scarce NHS resources should be targeted at those
patients whom it is most cost-effective to treat. Thus purchasers are
obliged to use both cost and outcome (effectiveness) data to
inform rationing choices.

If the choice is between therapies A and B with characteristics as
set out in Table 1, the EBM clinician concerned with effectiveness
alone would elect for therapy B, which produces eight additional
years of good quality life in comparison to therapy A. However, the
purchaser is interested in the 'biggest bang for the buck' and
therapy A is more cost-effective than therapy B. Put another way, if

Table 1. Rationing by effectiveness and efficiency

	Effectiveness (QALYs)*	Cost (£)	Cost-effectiveness (average)†
Therapy A	7	490	70
Therapy B	15	1,500	100

*QALYs: quality per adjusted life years
†Cost per QALY

the purchaser had a budget of £250,000 for this therapeutic area, therapy A is superior to therapy B as it produces over 3,571 QALYs compared to only 2,500 from funding therapy B.

This conflict between evidence-based medicine (whose advocates support the provision of the more effective but less cost-effective therapy B) and evidence-based purchasing (whose advocates support the provision of the more cost-effective but less effective therapy A) is the familiar clash between the individual ethic of the physician and the population ethic of the purchaser. Physicians, in principle, are trained to do their best for the individual patients in their care. The manager, in seeking the greatest population health gain from his or her budget, is seeking to get the physician to treat those patients who benefit most per unit of expenditure.

The tension between the population ethic of the manager and the individual ethic of the physician will always exist. What is required is that the relevant choice information is generated so that the parties can monitor each other's behaviour and induce greater account-ability. Given the poverty of the evidence base and the variation in the attributes of individual patients, physicians need and patients may benefit from some degree of discretion (or clinical autonomy). However, unfettered autonomy is unlikely to ensure that society's scarce health care resources are used efficiently.

Rationing efficiently and equitably

Over twenty years ago the American economist Victor Fuchs argued that rationing by efficiency considerations alone was an inadequate basis for choice. Choices in health care were and are determined by many social values including that of efficiency. Fuchs argued:[2]

> At the root of most of our major health problems are value choices. What kind of people are we? What kind of life do we want to lead?

What kind of society do we want to build for our children and grandchildren? How much weight do we want to put on individual freedom? How much to equality? How much to material progress? How much to the realm of the spirit? How important is our own health to us? How important is our neighbour's health to us? The answer we give to these questions, as well as the guidance we get from economies, will and should shape health care policy.

What social values, in addition to effectiveness and efficiency, are relevant for informing health care choices? There are a variety of equity arguments in the literature. For instance Williams[3] has explored the issue of intergenerational equity and the concept of the 'fair innings'. The social value he advocates is that each age cohort should have a 'fair innings' and this may necessitate the transfer of resources from the old to the young. In other words, to achieve a 'fair innings', the purchaser may direct resources away from the efficient treatment of the old and towards the inefficient treatment of the young. Grimley Evans opposes this position,[4] as does Harris (see Chapter 7), but does society?

The political issue is how society interprets equity. One element of social equity may be the 'fair innings' but this has to be determined by public debate and the elucidation of how much 'fair innings' redistribution is demanded by society. Different volumes of such redistribution will involve different amounts of opportunity cost and it would be useful to identify which of the elderly lose what interventions.

Another equity issue of concern to some societies is social class variations in health. A purchaser may wish to reduce the differences in the health of the social classes of the rich and the poor. He may, as a consequence, decide to purchase health care interventions which are not efficient but benefit the poor. Thus instead perhaps of targeting care efficiently at the rich, the purchaser may allocate resources cost ineffectively to improve the health of the poor and rescue the class health differential.

Whatever the equity targets desired by society, it is essential to identify them and monitor their opportunity cost in terms of health gains forgone due to inefficient but equitable rationing.

Rationing: national and local perspectives

The allocation of scarce NHS resources, that is rationing, will be informed by consideration of effectiveness (EBM), cost-effectiveness and equity. To ensure both the achievement of social priorities in rationing and the accountability of the rationers, clinical and non-clinical, the principles of rationing should be explicit not only in terms of efficiency and equity but also in terms of trade-offs; for example, how much efficiency is society prepared to forgo to achieve a 'fair innings', however defined?

Who should determine these principles? A public debate about rationing would be useful and a national priority-setting framework would seem appropriate. If local purchasers choose to ignore national guidelines their choices would be explicit and they would be accountable.

At present the problem is that there is no national framework for rationing and local NHS purchasers use different criteria with varying degrees of explicitness. Thus whilst Cambridge Health Authority refused to treat Child B on the basis of lack of effectiveness, other purchasers indicated they would have treated her. When she had had private therapy she was cared for until her death in a health authority neighbouring Cambridge. Other examples of variation in rationing criteria are interferon beta for multiple sclerosis patients and the availability of synthetic factor 8 for haemophiliacs. Within a National Health Service there is unequal access to therapy because of the absence of a national rationing framework and the reluctance of central government to make decision-makers accountable in terms of efficiency and equity.

Overview: rationing and elderly people

There is evidence of elderly people being deprived of efficient interventions[5] and if the purpose of the NHS is to use its budget to maximise improvements in the health status of the population, this is an inappropriate way to ration scarce resources. However, society may work to achieve goals other than mere efficiency and may be prepared to forgo the efficient production of health gains for elderly people in order to redistribute resources to the chronically ill young and give them a 'fairer innings'. The impact of the combined effects of increased longevity, technological change and public expectations may be that at last there is a public debate about how scarce NHS resources are allocated. It is impossible to treat all patients and it is inevitable that some potentially beneficial interventions will not be provided. The 'closet' discussion of rationing issues serves patients, taxpayers and society badly. With better definition of the principles and practices of rationing the NHS might, after 50 years, finally be organised to meet the 'needs' discussed by its founding fathers.

References

1   Sackett DL, Rosenberg WHC, Muir Gray JA, Haynes RB, Richardson WS. Evidence based medicine: what it is and what it isn't. *British Medical Journal* 1996; **312**: 71–2.

2   Fuchs V. *Who shall live?* New York: Basic Books, 1974: 148.

3   Williams A. The rationing debate: rationing health care by age: the case for. *British Medical Journal* 1997; **314**: 820–2.

4   Grimley Evans J. The rationing debate: rationing by age: the case against. *British Medical Journal* 1997; **314**: 822–5.

5   Maynard A. Prioritising health care: dreams and reality. In Malek M (ed). *Setting priorities in health care.* Wiley: Chichester, 1994.

4 | Advances in understanding the concept of biological ageing

Michael A Horan
Professor of Geriatric Medicine, University of Manchester

A precise explanation of what causes the ageing of an individual (biological ageing) and what processes bring it about is not yet possible, though we have strong evidence that they are in part genetically determined. Since life continues until a fatal event is encountered, an acceptable working definition of ageing is certain biological events occurring over time which impair the ability of an organism to withstand potentially fatal challenges and are associated with an increasing likelihood of death.

For evolutionary biologists, ageing may well have straightforward causes: the fading out of natural selection with age and the costs of long-term maintenance of the soma.[1] However, it does not follow from this that ageing is brought about by a single physiological mechanism, but by several, and these may differ between species. Hence, most contemporary discussions have abandoned the singular term in favour of the plural forms, ageing processes and ageing mechanisms. These underlying processes and their manifestations in the aged phenotype are modified throughout life by the effects of environmental factors (nutrition, radiation, injuries) and the legacy of past diseases, susceptibility to which is modified by stage of development[2] and genetic factors.

Physiological versus pathological ageing

The proposition that chronological age might be an inadequate measure of ageing was probably first introduced in Korenchevsky's influential book, *Physiological and pathological ageing.*[3] He was clearly concerned about how disease might obscure the effects of under-lying ageing processes and wrote: 'No human being has yet been identified whose old age, lifespan and death are physiologically normal. The aged individual is so subject to pathological defects that death as a natural biological phenomenon is yet beyond his reach'. He was obviously struck by the immense variation in anatomical, physiological and biochemical parameters seen in cross-sectional studies and noted that some very old people had values similar to those in young adults, while other old people had markedly lower values. Parameters with values close to the highest seen in the young were thought to define resistance to ageing, what Rowe and Kahn[4] would call 'successful ageing'. Successful ageing most likely reflects successful adaptations to age-specific losses and challenges. Those parameters with values close to the average for the young defined the condition typical for physiological old age (what Rowe and Kahn would call 'usual ageing'). Very low values indicated pathological old age (which might also be called 'unsuccessful ageing').

Korenchevsky's term 'physiological ageing' has now been replaced by 'biological ageing',[5] sometimes called 'functional ageing'. It follows that if the causes of pathological ageing could be prevented or cured, physiologically normal ageing would be the result. These ideas underpin the apophthegm, so commonly encountered in geriatric medicine texts, 'ageing is not disease and disease is not ageing': the ageing–disease dichotomy.

The ageing-disease dichotomy

Although it is practically useful to draw a clear distinction between ageing and disease, the basis on which this might be done lacks a clear scientific foundation[6] and it would be unwise to accept it uncritically. Earlier authors have expressed similar views.[7] On the basis of the age pattern of occurrence of diseases, they separated them into two groups: age-related diseases and age-dependent diseases (Table 1). If the pattern resembled that of the age-specific death rate, they were classed as age-dependent (and possibly involved ageing processes in their pathogenesis), whereas if the pattern differed, they were classed as age-related (and were unlikely to involve ageing processes). However, deaths from acute infections in old age, at least in the 1940s, also follow the age-dependent pattern,[8] but nobody would seriously propose that they emerge from ageing processes. Clearly, the relationship is much more complex.

Successful ageing

The idea of successful ageing referred to above now embraces not only the biological domain but also both cognitive and social

Table 1. Ageing and diseases (after Brody and Schneider[7])

Age-dependent (ageing involved)	Age-related (ageing not involved)
Acute myocardial infarction	Multiple sclerosis
Ischaemic heart disease	Motor neurone disease
Cerebrovascular disease	Gout
Diabetes mellitus type II	Peptic ulcer disease
Osteoporosis	Most cancers
Alzheimer's disease	
Parkinson's disease	
Prostate cancer	

domains.[9] In essence, it refers to the ability to use (coping) strategies to exploit reserve capacities fully, employ supportive measures and seek less demanding environments in order to achieve desirable goals, even in a setting in which a person's goals have had to be restructured.

Chronological age versus biological age

Most gerontologists do not accept chronological age (a linear function) as an adequate indicator of the extent of ageing because it is thought that individuals of the same species age at different rates. Furthermore, their preferred measure of the rate of ageing, the risk of dying, increases exponentially with time, and such a measure cannot be applied to individuals. Thus, it is not surprising that intense efforts have been made to identify a small number of measurable parameters that serve as markers for the rate of biological ageing,[4,10,11] so-called 'biomarkers of ageing'. None has yet been identified that performs better than chronological age. One explanation for the failure of this approach is that data analysis has relied on the inappropriate use of multiple regression.[12] Alternative approaches have not yet been established in terms of their utility for biological age calculation. The time-honoured approach is still being aggressively championed,[13–15] and equally aggressively opposed.[16,17]

Studies with experimental animals have been no more successful and the classical studies of Ganetzky and Flannagan[18] exemplify this. Studying ageing *Drosophila melanogaster*, they found that many physiological variables that decline with age play no causal role in the events leading to death. They went on to try to identify age-dependent physiological changes that occur later in genetically long-lived *Drosophila* than they do in short-lived ones. The *only* measure they found was the time taken for 10 out of 20 flies knocked to the bottom of a glass vial to leave the bottom of the vial, what they refer to as locomotor incapacitation. This phenomenon has obvious parallels with the medical concept of frailty.

Frailty

Frailty, like ageing, lacks a precise definition. We all use the word frequently and seem to imply concepts such as loss of vigour, weakness, fragility and vulnerability. Fried[19] adds to these the predisposition to adverse health outcomes like dependency, disability, falls, injuries, slow recovery, institutionalisation and death. Frail patients often complain of weakness and fatigue, poor appetite and weight loss and, when examined, are found to be thin, deconditioned and to have poor balance. Buchner and Wagner[20] consider that neurological, musculoskeletal and energy metabolism disorders are the most important. Speechley and Tinetti[21] attempted an empirical definition using factor analysis and proposed frailty as the possession of four or more of the features listed in Table 2. It is also argued that there is a precursor state of frailty that Speechley and Tinetti define as the possession of three of the factors listed in Table 2. Further, advanced frailty may well be simply a synonym for the syndrome of 'failure to thrive',[22] which is generally thought to be irreversible.

These ideas have been heavily championed in the US, as exemplified by a series of eight intervention trials funded by the National Institute on Ageing (FICSIT – Frailty and Injuries:

Table 2. Frailty factors (after Speechly and Tinetti, 1992[21])

Age > 80 years
Balance/gait abnormalities
Infrequent walking for exercise
Depression
Sedative use
Reduced strength in shoulders and/or knees
Lower limb disability
Near vision loss

Cooperative Studies of Intervention Technology).[23] We already know that substantial benefits may be gained from strength training, even in extremely old nursing home residents.[24]

The concept of frailty and its precursor state is attractive since it makes no assumptions about origins. It seems likely that intrinsic ageing, co-morbidity, environment and lifestyle factors all contribute. Further research should improve our understanding of the factors that constitute and predispose to frailty, some of which may be amenable to further therapeutic interventions.

Conclusion

The distinction between biological age and chronological age is probably valid but unproven. With more appropriate analytical techniques, a number of biomarkers will probably emerge that more or less efficiently predict the likelihood of death, though it is very likely that they will not have any simple or meaningful relationship to underlying ageing processes. The idea of lumping them together to characterise biological age is highly questionable. Furthermore, discovering a panel of biomarkers could well turn out to be disadvantageous, rather like the story of a man with a watch knowing the time but the man with two watches not being so sure.

To my mind, the most significant advance in this field has been the development of the concept of frailty. It appears to be valid and makes no theoretical assumptions about its origins. The identification of risk factors amenable to interventions holds out the possibility of desirable health gains for many older people. Biomarker research seems to offer little other than to provide spurious end-points against which to test interventions that might modify ageing, an objective that is likely to be socially divisive and ethically distasteful.

References

1 Rose MR. *Evolutionary biology of aging.* Oxford University Press, 1991: 164.
2 Barker DJP. *Mothers, babies, and disease in later life.* London: BMJ Publishing Group, 1994.
3 Korenchevsky V. *Physiological and pathological ageing.* Basel: Karger, 1961.
4. Rowe JW, Kahn RL. Human aging: usual and successful. *Science* 1987; **237**: 143–9.
5 Bellamy D. Assessing biological age: reality? *Gerontology* 1995; **41**: 322–4.

6   Horan MA, Pendleton N. Relationship between aging and disease. *Reviews in Clinical Gerontology* 1995; **5**: 125–41.

7   Brody JA, Schneider EL. Diseases and disorders of aging: a hypothesis. *Journal of Chronic Diseases* 1986; **39**: 871–6.

8   Dublin LI, Lotka AJ, Spiegelman M. *Length of life – a study of the life table*, Revised edition. New York: Ronald Press, 1949.

9   Baltes MM. Successful ageing. In: Ebrahim S, Kalache A (eds). *Epidemiology in old age*. London: BMJ Publishing Group, 1996: 162–8.

10 Ludwig FC, Smoke ME. The measurement of biological age. *Experimental Aging Research* 1980; **6**: 497–522.

11 Baker GT, Sprott RL. Biomarkers of aging. *Experimental Gerontology* 1988; **23**: 223–39.

12 Hochschild R. Improving the precision of biological age determinations. Part 1: A new approach to calculating biological age. *Experimental Gerontology* 1989; **24**: 289–300.

13 Dean W, Morgan RF. In defense of the concept of biological aging measurement – current status. *Archives of Gerontology and Geriatrics* 1988; **7**: 191–210.

14 Bulpitt CJ. Assessing biological age: practicality? *Gerontology* 1995; **41**: 315–21.

15 Galzigna L, Cecchettin M. A simple procedure for calculating biological age. *Gerontology* 1995; **41**: 325.

16 Adelman RC. Biomarkers of aging. *Experimental Gerontology* 1987; **22**: 227–9.

17 Costa PT, McCrae RR. Measures and markers of biological aging: 'a great clamoring... of fleeting significance'. *Archives of Gerontology and Geriatrics* 1988; **7**: 211–14.

18 Ganetzky B, Flanagan JR. On the relationship between senescence and age-related changes in two wild-type strains of *Drosophila melanogaster*. *Experimental Gerontology* 1978; **13**: 189–96.

19 Fried LP. Frailty. In: Hazzard WR, Bierman EL, Blass JP, Ettinger WH, Halter JB (eds). *Principles of geriatric medicine and gerontology*, 3rd edn. New York: McGraw-Hill, 1994: 1149–56.

20 Buchner DM, Wagner EH. Preventing frail health. *Clinics in Geriatric Medicine* 1992; **8**: 1–17.

21 Speechley M, Tinetti M. Falls and injuries in frail and vigorous community elderly persons. *Journal of the American Geriatrics Society* 1992; **39**: 46–52.

22 Sarkisian CA, Lachs MS. 'Failure to thrive' in older adults. *Annals of Internal Medicine* 1996; **124**: 1072–8.

23 Ory MG, Schlechtman KB, Miller P, *et al*. Frailty and injury in later life: the FICSIT trials. *Journal of the American Geriatrics Society* 1993; **41**: 283–96.

24 Hodes RJ. Frailty and disability: can growth hormone or other trophic agents make a difference? *Journal of the American Geriatrics Society* 1994; **42**: 1208–11.

5 | New technology and the aged patient

Sir Miles Irving
*Director, NHS Health Technology Programme and
Professor of Surgery, University of Manchester*

There is undoubtedly going to be in the future a whole range of new technologies relevant to the aged patient. As a surgeon, I think immediately of new operations. In my life, the importance of operations in enhancing quality of life and restoring independence has been quite outstanding, the most notable examples being joint replacements. The point has been made that even if you do not treat those who have had 'a good innings' it does not mean they are going to die soon afterwards. Many will continue to live with their disabilities and there is no doubt that hip replacement and other joint replacement surgery has the capacity to restore independence and dignity and therefore is highly cost-effective.

In the future there are certainly going to be new drugs, new devices, new instruments, new investigations and new services. All are open to use and abuse, and may cause benefit or harm, and it is these aspects that the National Health Service is addressing through the Research and Development Directorate in general and the Health Technology Programme in particular.

Health technology assessment (HTA)

Our official definition of HTA is the evaluation of health technologies in terms of effectiveness, costs and impact; so the points made by Alan Maynard (Chapter 3) about the need for a wider evaluation are very much taken into account. We cannot dissociate effectiveness from costs and impact and thus the evidence-based philosophy takes them into account. But what is the definition of a health technology? The NHS research and development programme's definition is a wide one: 'any procedure used by health professionals to promote health, to prevent and treat disease and to foster improved rehabilitation and long-term care'. All of these aspects are particularly relevant in the care of the aged patient.

Our definition covers both existing technologies and developing technologies, but because of the vast number involved we have to prioritise the need for assessment.

The benefits of HTA (which are now beginning to materialise from the NHS programme) will be to provide clinicians, managers and patients with the information needed to make decisions about the rational use of resources. I believe that the main drivers of HTA in the future will be the patients and consequently I believe that the next major task we have to undertake is the education of the public in the concepts of 'uncertainty' and 'evaluation'. It is going to be a big task but, nevertheless, we are already well on the way. However, it must be realised that the success of the Health Technology Programme, in the end, is not going to be in undertaking the evaluations as much as in delivering and implementing the results of evaluations.

What has been interesting about this programme so far is not only the result of the evaluations we have undertaken but the change in culture that has occurred, particularly in the health care professions, regarding the need for evaluation.

It is remarkable that it was only in 1992 that the realisation was forced on the health care professions that they ought to be looking at health technologies in a different light. It was Ian Chalmers' report to the Department of Health, *Assessing the effects of health technologies*,[1] which led to the setting up of the Standing Group on Health Technologies, and the Health Technology Programme. It pointed out that many widely used technologies ultimately have been shown to be ineffective or harmful. Equally, some technologies which were recognised as effective were being adopted only after unnecessary delays. Finally some new technologies were shown to have no advantage over existing simpler and cheaper alternatives. The latter is now quite obvious in many fields, particularly in surgical technologies. However, as Chalmers pointed out, in the case of the majority of technologies, we just do not know their efficacy, effectiveness and costs.

That message has been reinforced rather nicely by Davidson in the *Health Care Forum Journal*.[2] He points to what he calls 'technological cancer', which results from failure to excise outdated and inappropriate technologies from the practice of medicine, coupled with the unchecked growth of new technologies. He states that such 'cancer', if left untreated, can prove fatal to the health care system in which it grows. I think we have to take his somewhat cynical view seriously because currently there is indeed a tidal wave of new technologies.

Alan Maynard (Chapter 3) mentioned the introduction of interferon beta for the treatment of multiple sclerosis and pointed to the lack of evidence for its efficacy and effectiveness. There is now a Trial Development Group looking at this particular issue – and it is a major problem. It is said that if we allow the unchecked growth of interferon beta usage at the present time, it could take up to 30% of our total drug budget. Here is a powerful and expensive drug which appears to affect the pathological markers but not the rate of accumulation of disability of relapsing multiple sclerosis. It has not as yet undergone effective health technology assessment. It is not just interferon beta that is the problem; it is all the other candidate drugs that are coming over the horizon for this particular condition.

The work of the Health Technology Programme

So, we do have problems in current health care with the tidal wave of new technologies. What are we doing about it? The Standing Group on Health Technology (SGHT) and its panels are multi-disciplinary groups. The SGHT is responsible to the Central Research and Development Committee for health technology assessment. It advises the NHS on the following:

- Interventions that should be assessed as a priority.
- Very importantly, the control of unevaluated methods. We now have, through Executive Letters, the ability to say to purchasers 'This particular technology is being evaluated; do not use it outside trials.' To give one example of the effectiveness of this approach: laparoscopic excision of colorectal cancer is an untried technology. There is a funded trial on the way and we have been able to say to purchasers 'Do not purchase this technology outside the trial.' All the specialist surgical associations have given the same advice to their members. The result is that we have relatively tight control now on the use of that technology.
- We also advise on the emergence of new treatments and diagnostic methods arising from science and technology and – what is equally important – the development of new research methods to evaluate health practice; for many of the research methods we have at the present time are inappropriate for the evaluation of new health technologies.

The annual cycle of prioritisation and commissioning new

technologies is now entering into its fourth year. It starts with a widespread consultation process. However, we are still not getting from health care professionals in general, the public and other interested bodies sufficient suggestions about technologies that need evaluating. Although we are not actually short of suggestions there are obviously areas where we are deficient and we need advice from a wider background.

When new technologies, which are unevaluated, are suggested they go to one of five panels: Primary and Community Care, Pharmaceutical Panel, Acute Sector, Population Screening, and Diagnostics and Imaging. In these panels they are assessed and prioritised before going to the Standing Group. The Methodology Panel has a particular role in suggesting new methodologies for health technology assessment, and suggests how they might be related to the other projects that we support. The Standing Group then identifies each year about 20–30 topics, bands them according to urgency of need for assessment and then forwards them to the Commissioning Group. The research is commissioned, the proposals assessed and eventually the results obtained. This year we are starting to get results from the programme and they are beginning to feed back useful information and suggestions for other aspects that need study.

Factors that are considered when we prioritise a new technology for assessment are its impact on health, the likely level of demand, risks or disadvantages to the patients, the NHS, the country, and the cost. We also take account of the feasibility of a useful assessment being achieved (if we do not think an assessment is feasible, obviously it is not worth doing), the likely impact of an assessment on practice and also what is going on in the way of similar studies elsewhere at home and overseas. In 1996 the organisation of the HTA programme was moved out of the Department of Health into a separate institution which has been contracted to undertake the work. The body concerned has been designated as the National Co-ordinating Centre for Health Technology Assessment, which is primarily at Southampton University but is supported by York University. It is to this Centre that suggestions for HTA topics should now be sent.

Our first priority setting exercise received 1,382 suggestions about technologies that people were using for which they felt there was uncertainty – and surely that number tells a story in itself. These suggestions were referred to the relevant panels, who each prioritised five high priority technologies together with another 15–20 in urgent need of assessment and referred them to the

Standing Group. The SGHT, after considering all submissions, identified 26 topics for assessment in rank order out of the 83 forwarded to them by the panels.

In the second year, the number of suggestions for assessment had fallen but nevertheless was large and the process was repeated. About one in four of these suggestions was worked up into a vignette; 60 recommendations were made to the Standing Group; and 41 were prioritised. In the third year we prioritised 66. I believe that this programme is helping to fulfil Archie Cochrane's original suggestion that effective health care should be based on hard evidence (preferably from randomised trials) that the use of each technology either alters the natural history of disease or otherwise benefits many patients at a reasonable cost.

By and large, we use two research methodologies to obtain our results. One is systematic reviews of existing evidence and the second is primary research, preferably where possible with randomised controlled trials (RCTs), but including observational studies as well. We also have two other main activities which are currently well on the way. The first is an inventory of all health technologies. This is being accumulated by the Wessex Institute and will give us an idea of the cost, the extent of the use, variations in use and known information on cost-effectiveness of all technologies used by the NHS. This should enable us to identify large areas of NHS activity for which there had been no scientific evaluation of cost-effectiveness. The other activity is forecasting, that is horizon-scanning for new and emerging technologies.

By 1996 the Health Technology Programme had funded in the region of 90 topics. This figure has now risen to 102. The first results we are receiving are the systematic reviews and they are likely to have a significant impact on health practice. The first major topic (launched at a press conference at the Royal College of Surgeons in February 1997) relates to the efficacy of screening for prostate cancer, but there are a large number of topics currently being peer-reviewed which will soon be ready for release.

Screening for prostate cancer

This topic was also the subject of a Canadian review, in 1995, which evaluated the benefits, health effects and costs of screening for cancer of the prostate.[3] Prostate-specific antigen (PSA) screening was a new technology introduced without evaluation in 1990. Its use in Canada increased tenfold over the ensuing years and, as a result, radical prostatectomy increased threefold between 1986 and 1993. But there is very little evidence for the value of doing radical prostatectomy. There have been no randomised control trials of sufficient size to judge the efficacy of this particular operation. The result has been enormous practice variation.

Practice variation is now recognised as a major problem in modern health care. Take, for example, Scandinavia, a set of countries with an established scientific tradition and good health care standards. If you have cancer of the prostate in Scandinavia, your treatment depends not on the scientific evidence but on which country you live in. In Denmark only about 10% of surgeons believe radical prostatectomy to be an established and effective treatment and a few more believe it is actually safe. But in Finland and Norway, some 60% of surgeons believe it to be a safe and effective treatment. In Sweden the percentage is a bit lower but not as low as in Denmark.[4] This confusion over the status of any treatment represents the problems of an unevaluated technology.

This same uncertainty exists for virtually all the common operations. For many conditions the treatment you get depends not on the scientific evidence but where you live. According to the Canadian review, the benefit resulting from surgery – radical prostatectomy – is probably in the order of one cancer prostate death avoided for every 100 operations but certainly never more than 7%. Bearing in mind that there is a mortality from the diagnostic prostatic biopsy and bearing in mind the mortality of radical prostatectomy can be up to 2%, then the gains look slim. Add to this the morbidity in terms of incontinence, which can be up to 20%, and the morbidity in terms of impotence, in the region of 70–80%; one can see that PSA screening of adult asymptomatic men is screening for a disease that we do not know how to treat.

Other HTA topics relating to the aged patient

In looking at cancer of the prostate we have addressed one major issue relevant to the aged. What other priorities have been put forward from the HTA programme that specifically relate to the aged? In the 1993 priorities we funded four projects on stroke rehabilitation. We have also studied hip replacement and prostheses, pressure sore management and community provision of hearing aids. In 1994, we looked at comparison of new and established treatments for benign prostatic hyperplasia, the use of laxatives in the elderly, management of hip fractures in fit patients, evaluation of rehabilitation of elderly patients and hearing loss in the over-60s.

In 1995 we prioritised evaluation of the effectiveness of discharge arrangements for elderly patients, treatment for glaucoma and geriatrician intervention following fracture for elderly patients. Similar concern with technologies relevant to the aged can be seen in the 1996 priorities.

Conclusion

What we have achieved so far is the easy bit. The problem we face now is disseminating the results and putting them into practice. A plan has been put forward for dissemination which recognises that we are going to need different routes for dissemination of different aspects of the programme. Screening for fragile X, which has just been the subject of a systematic review, is unlikely to need widespread dissemination. In contrast the recommendations for prostate cancer screening are of widespread concern, as will be those for the use of laxatives for the elderly. So routes of dissemination will involve Regional R&D Directors, publications, Executive Letters, College guidelines and the National Research Register to mention a few. One of our most effective techniques is the *Effective Health Care Bulletin.* Existing issues deal with such topics as preventing falls and subsequent injury in older people, whilst an issue of *Effectiveness Matters* deals with influenza vaccination and older people.

In conclusion, any procedure contemplated for use in the NHS should first be evaluated and, if it is not useful, rejected, leaving only those that are useful to be taken up. Our problem is that so many unevaluated technologies go round the route of the so-called 'evaluation bypass', in which individual enthusiasms, convictions, and particularly in surgery, commercial pressures are the principal factors governing acceptance. We have to discipline ourselves by following the evaluation path. I believe that the rationing agenda can, up to a point, be put on the back boiler, if we all try to make sure that what we do is effective and cost-effective. Our goal is a health technology programme that will bring us forward to practise evidence-based health care.

References

1   Chalmers I. Assessing the effects of health technologies. 10/92/FM. Department of Health, 1992.
2   Davidson SN. Technology, medicine and health, Part 4. *Healthcare Forum Journal* 1995; **38** (2): 52–8.

3   Health Technology Assessment Council of Quebec. Screening for cancer of the prostate. An evaluation of benefits, unwanted health effects and costs. Quebec: HTA Council of Quebec, August 1995.

4   Jonsson PM, Danneskiold-Samsoe B, Heggestad T, Iversen P, Leisti S. Management of early prostatic cancer in the Nordic countries: variations in clinical policies and physicians' attitudes toward radical treatment options. *International Journal of Technology Assessment in Health Care* 1995; **11**: 66–78.

6 | Making rational use of resources

Chris Ham
Professor of Health Policy and Management and Director of the
Health Services Management Centre, University of Birmingham

My starting point in discussing the rational use of resources is that priority setting in health care is inevitable. Resources will never be sufficient to meet all demands, and choices therefore have to be made about the priority to be attached to different services and patients. In the National Health Service (NHS), these choices have in the past been mainly the responsibility of clinicians. Doctors have rationed resources in a variety of ways by placing patients on waiting lists for non-urgent treatment, but also by deciding which patients should receive access to specialist services such as dialysis and transplants.

One of the changes brought about by the NHS reforms is that rationing, a word I shall use as a synonym for priority setting, has become more transparent. This has resulted from the separation of purchaser and provider responsibilities and the requirement that health authorities specify in their contracts with NHS trusts the services they wish to purchase. In addition, patients are no longer willing to accept that doctor knows best and are increasingly prepared to question and challenge medical decisions. Implicit rationing is therefore becoming explicit and this in turn is generating a wider public debate about health services funding and priorities.

The challenge of rationing is not confined to the United Kingdom. At a recent international conference in Stockholm, delegates from many countries gathered to discuss how priorities are set and the development of more systematic approaches to this task. Of particular interest in this respect are the initiatives taken in Oregon, the Netherlands, New Zealand and Sweden. Policy-makers in these systems have established national committees to advise on priority setting and to analyse the issues involved. The UK government has only belatedly chosen to follow this example and until now has relied mainly on health authorities and GP fundholders to take decisions on priorities.

Government policy on rationing

The Conservative government's views on rationing were set out in the 1996 White Paper on the future of the NHS.[1] The White Paper reviewed the evidence that pressures on the NHS were increasing because of demographic changes, advances in health care tech-nology and rising public expectations. It concluded that there were no reasons to believe that these pressures could not be accom-modated with a commitment to increase health service expendi-ture in real terms each year. In putting forward this argument, the Conservative government maintained that to draw up a national list of services to be funded Oregon-style was not appropriate in the UK. Rather, the emphasis should be placed on using NHS resources on treatments of proven effectiveness and ensuring that new technologies were properly evaluated before being adopted.

A number of questions arise from the White Paper. First, what-ever the future may hold, the NHS is currently under enormous pressure and rationing is an everyday occurrence. In no particular order, this pressure derives from:

- an increase in emergency medical admissions to acute hospitals
- a concern to reduce waiting times for non-emergency treatment
- shortages of intensive care facilities
- the availability of expensive new drugs
- increasing demands in the mental health field both for specialist services and for community care
- the growing number of elderly people in the population in need of continuing care

In my work with health authorities, it has become clear that extremely difficult choices now face the NHS. In some inner London health authorities, for example, consideration is being given to radical cuts in budgets and services in 1997/8 to enable budgets to be balanced. The debate about rationing is not there-fore a hypothetical argument about some possible future, it is an immediate challenge.

Second, the White Paper does not specify the level of growth in NHS resources that will be made available in future. While the government made a welcome commitment to increase spending in real terms, the historical record suggests that there is a world of difference between annual increases in expenditure of 3% in real terms and 0.3%. The pressures under which the NHS is operating reflect the government's decision to curb the budget in 1996/7 to little more than is needed to allow for NHS inflation. The effect is that health authorities have little room for manoeuvre. Unless there is a return to the more generous levels of funding provided in the early 1990s, then the gap between demand and supply will widen. In a climate of tax resistance and public expenditure constraints, the prospects are not encouraging.

Third, it has to be questioned whether a national list of services to be funded is the only alternative to the existing policy of muddling through. The experience of countries that have adopted a more systematic approach to priority setting indicates that a range of methods has been used and defining a set of core services is in fact the exception rather than the rule. This is illustrated by New Zealand where the government-appointed Core Services Committee declined to draw up a menu of services to be provided in that country's health services and instead initiated a programme of work focusing on how particular services might be provided more effectively. This included developing guidelines for the delivery of care and criteria to determine access to elective surgery designed to give priority to the most urgent cases and to replace waiting lists with a booking system.

The experience of countries like New Zealand that have adopted a more systematic approach indicates what a more rational approach to priority setting might involve. To begin with, it demands a significant and sustained investment in work on clinical effectiveness and cost-effectiveness. In this respect, at least, the UK has made a promising start. Specifically, the work initiated by Michael Peckham as part of the Department of Health's research and development programme means that there is now a good basis on which to build.[2] This is illustrated by the activities of the NHS Centre for Reviews and Dissemination, the Cochrane Centre and the investment made in health technology assessment. In their different ways, these initiatives are focusing attention on clinical effectiveness and providing purchasers with information they can use in their negotiations with providers.

Lessons from abroad

Beyond this, what is also needed is national leadership and an acknowledgement on the part of politicians that priority setting does present a challenge. It is here that UK health ministers can learn most from their counterparts elsewhere. As an example, in

the Netherlands, the current health minister, Dr Borst-Eilers, a
clinician by background, is taking forward the work initiated by the
Dunning Committee in 1991. The Committee's framework for
thinking about priorities is illustrated in Fig 1.[3] Four tests were
proposed by the Dunning Committee for determining whether a
service should be funded. These involve asking whether a service is
necessary from the community's point of view, whether it is
effective and efficient, and whether it could be left to personal
responsibility. Services that pass these tests are included in the
health benefits package. Those that do not are excluded.

In the Netherlands, the government has reviewed whether a
number of services should be funded using this framework. In the
case of in-vitro fertilisation (IVF), three cycles of treatment are
funded but if these are not successful then further treatment is a
matter of personal responsibility. This decision is based in part on
evidence that if IVF is unsuccessful after three cycles of treatment
then it is unlikely to be effective. Another example is dental care
for adults, which is excluded from funding on the basis that it is
affordable and should be paid for directly by individuals. The
health minister also initiated discussion on contraceptive pills,

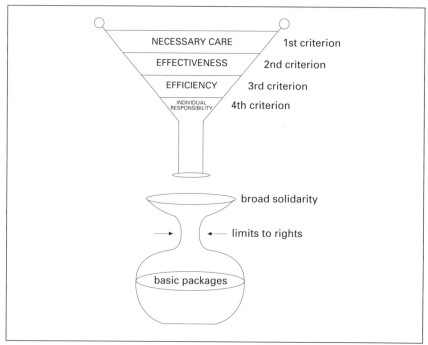

Fig 1. *The Dunning Committee's four sieves for health services*

arguing that these should be paid for privately as they were cheap and freely available. However, this proposal was withdrawn after opposition from women's groups and others.

Of increasing importance in the Netherlands has been the attempt to involve clinicians in thinking about priority setting. Alongside the national debate on funding services such as IVF, adult dental care and contraceptives, effort has been put into work with the health care professions on waiting list priorities and on the development of guidelines and protocols. This has been stimulated by recognition that making more effective use of resources involves changing clinical practice patterns. The involvement of doctors, nurses and other professionals is therefore essential. In addition, research has been set in hand to evaluate the effectiveness of both existing and new health care technologies. The most recent report from the Dutch government emphasises too the need to involve and inform patients' organisations about the appropriate use of health care services.[4] This is part of an overall strategy to ensure that resources are deployed in the most cost-effective manner.

One of the lessons from experience in New Zealand and the Netherlands is the need for action at different levels. National leadership must go hand in hand with local action and with full participation by the health care professions and others. Part of the rationale behind this is that it will help in promoting greater public understanding of the dilemmas involved in rationing. Put another way, health literacy, to borrow the term coined by a former health secretary in the UK, will be enhanced if lay people, doctors, managers and politicians are involved. Yet, as the Stockholm conference on priority setting demonstrated, this is necessarily a long-term process and requires a sustained effort over a period of time before the effects are felt. Indeed, while some progress has been made in making available more information on clinical effectiveness to inform decisions on priorities, much less has been done to engage the public in the debate.

Lessons from long-term care of the elderly

What are the risks in not following the example of the Netherlands, New Zealand and other countries? These risks are perhaps best illustrated by what has happened recently in the field of long-term care for elderly people. The progressive withdrawal of the NHS from the provision of long-term care has meant that responsibility has passed to local authorities and to those requiring care and their families. As the Ombudsman's inquiry into the Leeds case shows,[5] this means that some people are not receiving care and are having to pay for it personally. This situation has arisen not through open debate and explicit policy-making but by stealth.

As a result of the Ombudsman's report, the Conservative government was forced to act and required health authorities and local authorities to draw up local policies to clarify responsibilities for continuing care. In some cases this entails health authorities contracting for additional services in their area in order to meet their obligations. In addition, the government has published proposals for the future of long-term care which make it clear that comprehensive state-funded services are not an option and that the main priority is being attached to the development of private insurance schemes which enable elderly people and their families to protect their assets.[6]

The fate of long-term care serves as a cautionary tale. If politicians are either unwilling or unable to acknowledge the challenges of rationing or priority setting, then other services will be affected in the same way. This has already started to happen in the case of dentistry and the growing gap between demand and supply in health care could affect mainstream services in a similar way. For example, if acute hospitals focus on treating emergency admissions at the expense of patients with non-urgent conditions, the funding of these conditions will have to come from private sources. This will result in increasing inequity but there may be no alternative in a situation in which public funding is highly constrained.

To make this point is to suggest that the change of government in May 1997 will not eliminate the rationing dilemma. The Labour government's policy on the NHS envisages no additional funding beyond the plans already announced. Some additional resources may be released for patient care by cutting back on bureaucracy but the sums involved are not likely to be sufficient to deal with the pressures currently in the system, let alone to fund new technologies in the future. At a time when Labour is seeking to shed its 'tax and spend' image, the prospects for NHS funding are not rosy. Indeed, Labour politicians appear just as reluctant to grasp the nettle of health care rationing as their opponents. To be sure, Labour has promised to establish a Royal Commission to investigate long-term care, but not to examine the rationing of other services. With some independent analysts challenging the view that the NHS is underfunded,[7] there are indeed serious obstacles to the development of a real debate about these issues.

References

1   Secretary of State for Health. *The National Health Service. a service with ambitions.* London: The Stationery Office, 1996.

2   NHS Executive. *Promoting clinical effectiveness.* Department of Health, 1996.

3   Government Committee on Choices in Health Care. *Report.* Rijswijk: Ministry of Welfare, Health and Cultural Affairs, 1991.

4   Borst-Eilers E. *Medical technology assessment and efficiency in health care.* Rijswijk: Ministry of Health, Welfare and Sport, 1996.

5   Health Service Commissioner. *Failure to provide long term NHS care for a brain-damaged patient,* Second Report for Session 1993–94. London: HMSO, 1994.

6   Secretary of State for Health. *A new partnership for care in old age.* London: HMSO, 1996.

7   Dixon J, Harrison A, New B. Is the NHS under funded? *British Medical Journal* 1997; **314**: 58–61.

7 | Are moral claims age-relative?

John Harris
Sir David Alliance Professor of Bioethics and Director of Institute for Medicine, Law and Bioethics, University of Manchester

An important question that must be settled before anything useful can be said about the values that should inform and indeed govern our attitudes to older people, and indeed to all of us as we age, is the question of whether or not people's legitimate moral claims are age-relative in any way.[1] By legitimate moral claims I mean a person's claims or entitlements to the concern, respect and protection of the community and of other individuals as expressed in three main ways:

1. In the form of legal protections whether these take the form of express statutory entitlements or more vague protections in the form perhaps of common law rights or rights protected by international conventions to which nations states are signatories.
2. In the form of entitlements to access to public resources or services.
3. In the form of less tangible expressions of concern, respect and protection in the form of family ties, friendship, community and basic civility.

Age-relative moral claims

There are three obvious ways in which it might be thought that moral claims could be age-relative. One is that they might be thought to vary with elapsed time, that they might diminish (or increase) in proportion to the amount of lifetime an individual had experienced or 'consumed'.[2] The second way in which moral claims might be thought to be age-relative concerns not lifetime lived, but lifetime in prospect. It is often thought that moral claims vary with life expectancy, in proportion to the amount of lifetime an individual has left or (more likely) is reasonably expected to have left. While this will always be related to elapsed time it may also arise through illness, injury or indeed, genetic constitution.

Finally, many think that moral claims are legitimately varied by quality of life considerations, for example that people with very poor quality of life are not worth (or are worth less than) the expenditure of health care resources.[3]

Quality, quantity and life expectancy considerations are all combined of course in the notorious QALY (quality adjusted life year) and related methods of prioritising resources for health care.[4] Elapsed time on the other hand features in accounts that use some concept of a 'fair innings' or 'reasonable lifespan' approach.[5] All of these accounts reflect significant concerns about the justice of ignoring quantity and quality of life considerations when considering entitlements. However, this chapter will articulate an alternative approach to these issues.

Another increasingly popular suggestion is that an individual's lifestyle choices may affect his or her moral claims or entitlements. This can happen in two main ways which I shall call *health-related* and *wealth-related* choices.

Health-related choices

Throughout a person's life he or she will make many choices and do many things which impact upon his or her health state and life expectancy. These will include choices about diet, drug and alcohol use and abuse, exercise and fitness, choice of domicile (cities are dangerous places – pollution or violent crime abounds, the south of Italy is well known to be more conducive to longevity than the north of England), choice of occupation (occupational risk and health) and indeed sexual habits and practices (numbers of partners, methods of contraception or lack of them etc). The list could continue almost indefinitely but there is an increasingly vocal school of thought which suggests that people be held responsible for adverse health that is wholly or partially attributable to their own voluntary choices.[6]

Wealth-related choices

Similarly, an individual will make what I call 'wealth-related' choices; choices which determine what disposable resources are available to palliate infirmity, support health care and retirement or old age. Such choices will include decisions to spend or save at various points in life, decisions to insure against various risks or certainties and, decisions (like the decision to have children) which may be calculated to reduce resources available for self-support or, under another model of the function of children, to provide support in old age.[7]

Some of the bases for an age-related approach to moral claims or entitlements and some of the other considerations like 'quality of life' and 'lifestyle choices' which relate crucially to age or life expectancy have been noted above and their importance and attraction have been acknowledged without any attempt to estab-lish either their importance or their attraction. This is because there is a need to establish what the alternative position might be, a position which has, perhaps surprisingly, been much less widely articulated or disseminated. We will call it, for want of a more appropriate title, 'the anti-ageist argument'.

The anti-ageist argument

One way of formulating the ideas that lie behind opposition to so-called *ageism* has been stated thus:

> All of us who wish to go on living have something that each of us values equally although for each it is different in character, for some a much richer prize than for others, and we none of us know its true extent. This thing is of course 'the rest of our lives'. So long as we do not know the date of our deaths then for each of us the 'rest of our lives' is of indefinite duration. Whether we are 17 or 70, in perfect health or suffering from a terminal disease we each have the rest of our lives to lead. So long as we each fervently wish to live out the rest of our lives, however long that turns out to be, then if we do not deserve to die, we each suffer the same injustice if our wishes are deliberately frustrated and we are cut off prematurely.[8]

An important element of an anti-ageist position expressed in this way is that it links discrimination on the basis of elapsed lifetime, to discrimination on the basis of life expectancy. These are not of course necessarily linked. Some people have defended what might be termed a 'fair innings argument' which we have already noted.[9] This suggests that people are entitled to every opportunity to live a fair lifespan – perhaps the traditional three score years and ten. Up to that point they have equal entitlement to health care, beyond the fair innings they are given very low priority. This argument is tempting because it explains the strong intuition people have that there is something wrong with treating the claims of an octo-genarian and those of a 20-year-old as equal. However, the fair innings argument has a number of defects. It assumes that the value of a life is to be measured in units of lifetime, the more the better up to a certain point but thereafter extreme discounting begins. The problem is that people value particular events within their life disproportionately to the time required to experience those events. Although the fair innings argument gives great importance to a life having shape and structure, these things are again not necessarily only achieved within a particular time-span. On the fair innings argument Nelson Mandela's entitlement to life-saving care from the community was over before he left Victor Verster Prison; the long road to freedom would have ended before Mandela's release. And it is not only for such as Mandela that the most important part of their life might well begin after a so-called 'fair innings' had been achieved.[10]

Without the vast detail of each person's life and their hopes and aspirations within that detail, we cannot hope to do justice between lives. The only sensible alternative is, arguably, to count each life for one and none for more than one, whatever the differences in age and in other quality considerations.

It is this outlook that explains why murder is always wrong and wrong to the same degree. When you rob someone of life you take from them not only all they have but all they will ever have; it is a difference in degree so radical that it makes for a difference in the quality of the act. However, the wrongness consists in taking from them something that they want. That is why voluntary euthanasia is no more wrong than suicide (although it may be bad policy) and murder is our paradigm of a wrongful act.

Those who believe in discriminating in favour of the young or against the old must believe that in so far as murder is an injustice it is less of an injustice to murder the old than the young and since they also believe that life years are a commodity like any other[11] it is clear that in robbing people of life you take less from them the less life expectancy they have. This is of course directly contrary to the way in which the common law tradition has viewed the wrong of ending life prematurely. As Mr Justice Mars Jones said in his judgement in a 1986 case:

> However gravely ill a man may be ... he is entitled in our law to every hour ... that God has granted him. That hour or hours may be the most precious and most important hours of a man's life. There may be business to transact, gifts to be given, forgiveness to be made, 101 bits of unfinished business which have to be concluded.[12]

The age-concern principle

If we try to derive from the anti-ageist argument an appropriate guiding principle, perhaps the following has some plausibility:

an individual's entitlement to the concern, respect and protection of the community does not vary with age or life expectancy.[13]

This principle has, I hope, a certain degree of what might be called 'epigrammatic validity'.[14] Clearly this principle is itself the application of a more general principle. That more general principle, which is clearly a principle of equality, may be taken as asserting that each person is entitled to the same concern, respect and protection of society as is accorded to any other person in the community. The principle of equality has the advantage of very wide appeal and acceptance, and versions of it are enshrined in many national constitutions throughout the world[15] and in various declarations of human rights.[16] The age-concern principle reminds us that the principle of equality applies as much in the face of discrimination on the basis of chronological age or life expectancy as it does to discrimination on the basis of gender, race and other arbitrary features.[17]

The age-concern principle, like many another moral principles, derives from (hopefully) convincing moral arguments. It sums up those arguments and presents their conclusions in a form which also acquires an independent resonance and appeal. This independent resonance and appeal derives in part from the principle's reflection of a pre-existing and accepted morality, in part from the ways in which it extends or makes clearer the application and relevance of that morality and partly from what I have termed its 'epigrammatic validity', from the way in which the power of the language in which it is expressed adds to its appeal. The strength of a clearly articulated principle which is resonant enough to be inspiring, and at the same time firmly grounded in established moral theory, custom and practice, is that it could inform and guide a community's approach to a broad range of legislative, policy and funding initiatives.

Can we be confident, however, that the age-concern principle is reasonably well grounded in moral theory, custom and practice? Where indeed do such principles come from?

Moral principles are not just plucked from the air,[18] but nor are they derived from unassailable premises or immutable absolutes. They articulate central elements of a shared morality. Like the 'ten commandments' they remind us of that morality and our commitment to it, and like the famous commandments they require interpretation.[19] Indeed it is their generality and their susceptibility to interpretation in the light of changing conditions, values and attitudes that is their strength. The Constitution of the United

States of America, for example, is constantly reinterpreted in the light of changing attitudes and values in the community.[20]

However, moral principles also differ from commandments in important ways. Unlike commandments they do not attempt self-justification, they do not purport to explain *why* they ought to be accepted. So, when we articulate a moral principle we are in a sense reminding ourselves of what we believe to be an important part of the morality we already accept. Moreover we hope and expect that others will share both the morality and the principles derived from it. We should follow the principle *because* we accept the morality, but the principle cannot give us *reasons for* accepting the morality.

When we encounter a principle we need first to reflect on our morality to see whether and how the principle fits with it. We then need to explore the consequences of accepting the principle to see whether we can adhere to it consistently with other moral beliefs we share and wish to retain. If the principle can be applied consistently with our general morality this is an added recommendation; if not, we have to choose whether to abandon the principle or abandon the elements of our morality which are not consistent with it.[21] When we recommend a principle to others we hope that they will go through the same process and that on reflection they will find not only that our principle is consonant with their existing morality but also that it extends that morality in ways which appeal to the very values that morality enshrines and expresses.

When, for example, Mr Justice Mars Jones suggested in his judgement that 'however gravely ill a man may be ... he is entitled in our law to every hour ... that God has granted him', he was articulating not only a rule of law, but a principle of morality. Indeed, the common law of England, from which this rule derives, is, in large measure, the systematisation of a shared, a common morality. In reminding us of the protections that the common law affords even to those terminally ill, Mars Jones J was also inviting us to apply that morality consistently to a hard case; a case that challenges both our morality and our moral psychology by presenting an apparent conflict between our instinctive reactions and our reflective morality.[22] In formulating the appropriate principle he is recommending a resolution of that tension.

Does our morality imply the age-concern principle?

There is a strong presumption in our society, and indeed in most others, that a person's moral claims derive from their dignity and standing as a human person and are not dependent on any more arbitrary or particular features. It is this generality that is found in almost all declarations of, or conventions on, human rights. However, this leaves immense room for manoeuvre in particular cases. Many legal systems for example give reduced legal protections to newborn infants.[23] If we extend our thoughts to political rights and liberties then we find a fairly massive consensus that these apply progressively through late childhood and early adolescence and reach their full flower only with the age of majority. At the other end of life it is not uncommon to find progressive disabilities from a compulsory age of retirement from employment to restrictions on travel and access to medical treatment.

However, the principle that an individual's entitlement to the concern, respect and protection of the community does not vary with age or life expectancy accords well with our general view that it is human persons who matter morally. More particularly that their claims on one another derive from their status as beings of a particular sort and not from contingent features of their lives like age, life expectancy or quality of life no more than from gender nor race.

The task must be to work through the consequences of this principle in particular cases. For example, in the case of prioritising scarce medical resources or scarce employment opportunities on the one hand or, on the other, if we are to include consideration of the justice of age-related disabilities at all stages of life, the case for example of the justice of denying the franchise to competent individuals below the age of majority. If we do so we may find that this society and many others do not consistently apply the very principles that underpin and express their morality.

Public policy

To reinforce the message delivered by so doing, it might well be instructive to reveal the obverse of the same coin. This might include demonstrating the values a society would have to embrace, or at least accept if it is to countenance age-related variance of moral entitlements. One of these is implicit in the judgement of Mars Jones J we have already noted. It is that a society which accords lower priority in the allocation of resources for health care to the old or those with reduced life expectancy is saying, in effect, that their lives are less worth saving, in short, are less valuable. If the right or good done in saving or preserving a life is the less, then so is the wrong done in taking it; which would make, for example, the crime of murder inevitably less serious when the victims are old or terminally ill.

This may be an undesirable message to deliver for public policy as well as for moral reasons. In other words even those who are not convinced that the moral arguments for insisting on the equal moral standing of the old are compelling, and who believe the aged to have reduced moral entitlements, might think that the message delivered by the corollary of that view was a dangerous one to brute abroad in a civilised society. The systematic dis-valuing of the old, or those with life-threatening illness, might have a corrosive effect on social morality and community relations more generally. It might for example lead to an increasing tolerance of the idea that any and all resources, or even care, devoted to the old or those with life-threatening disease was a waste of time, money and emotion. Even if this were the right view to take, the sort of society that implemented such views at the level of policy might be increasingly one in which others would feel threatened and uneasy. Moreover, once the old, however defined, had been ruled out of account the middle-aged would become the old. They would after all have greater elapsed time 'in the bank' and shorter life expectancy ahead, than the rest of society and the cycle of argument and discrimination would have a tendency to extend indefinitely, a tendency moreover which it would be difficult to restrain.

If we were to attempt to translate this into a principle for the allocation of public resources to health care we might do worse than the following: the principal objective of a public health care system should be to protect the life and health of each citizen impartially and to offer beneficial health care on the basis of individual need, so that each has an equal chance of flourishing to the extent that their personal health status permits. This equal chance of flourishing should be available regardless of such arbitrary features as race, gender, religious belief, skin colour, age or life expectancy.[24]

Endnotes

1 Much of the stimulus for this paper derives from my participation in the Millennium Papers project for Age Concern and my Chairmanship of their working party on 'Values, Attitudes and Lifestyles'. My indebtedness to all the members of this working party, and especially to its rapporteur Justine Burley, is substantial.

2 See, for example, Norman Daniels *Justice and justification* (Cambridge

University Press, Cambridge; 1996) and Ronald Dworkin *Life's dominion* (London: Harper Collins, 1993).

3 See A Sen 'What is Equality?' in S Darwall (ed) *Equal freedom* (Michigan: Michigan University Press, 1995) and his 'Equality of what?' in S McMurrin (ed) *Equality, liberty and law* (Cambridge: Cambridge University Press, 1987).

4 See, for example, Alan Williams 'Economics, society and health care ethics' in Raanan Gillon (ed) *Principles of Medical Ethics* (Chichester: John Wiley & Sons, 1994) and John Harris 'QALYfying the value of life' in *Journal of Medical Ethics* 1987; **13**: 117–23.

5 See, for example, Norman Daniels *Justice and justification* (Cambridge: Cambridge University Press, 1996, Chapter 12); Ronald Dworkin *Life's Dominion* (London: Harper Collins, 1993, 87–89, 99); and John Harris *The value of life* (London: Routledge & Kegan Paul, 1985, Chapter 5).

6 See Norman Daniels *Seeking fair treatment* (Oxford: Oxford University Press, 1995); and Ronald Dworkin 'Justice in the distribution of health care' in *McGill Law Review* 1993; **38**: 883–98.

7 See GA Cohen 'On the currency of egalitarian justice' in *Ethics* 1990; 906–44; Ronald Dworkin 'What is Equality? Part II' *Philosophy and Public Affairs* 1981; and Ronald Dworkin 'Foundations of liberal equality' in S Darwall (ed) *Equal freedom* (Michigan: Michigan University Press, 1995).

8 John Harris *The value of life* (London: Routledge and Kegan Paul, 1985: 89). I would now drop the word 'fervently' from this statement of the argument against ageism. Since we cannot sensibly measure degrees of desire it is enough that the individual wants their life to continue given that they understand the costs to themselves and others of granting this wish and accept those costs.

9 See, for example, Daniel Callahan *What kind of life: the limits of medical progress (New York: Simon and Schuster,* 1990).

10 I cannot hope here to do justice to the complexity of the arguments surrounding fair innings, and other value of life considerations. I discuss them in detail in *The value of life* (London: Routledge and Kegan Paul, 1985) and in 'More and better justice' in Sue Mendus and Martin Bell (eds) *Philosophy and medical welfare* (Cambridge: Cambridge University Press, 1988: 75–97).

11 Kappel K and Sandoe P 'QALYs. Age and fairness' in *Bioethics* 1992; **6**(4): 314–5.

12 *R v. Carr, Sunday Times,* 30 November 1986.

13 I first articulated this principle in 'Ethical issues in geriatric medicine' in Tallis R, Fillet H and Brocklehurst JC (eds) *Textbook of geriatric medicine and gerontology,* 5th edn (London: Churchill Livingstone, 1998, in press).

14 I owe this phrase to Frank Cioffi.

15 For example, those of the United States of America and France.

16 For example, the Universal Declaration of Human Rights (Articles 1 and 2) and the European Convention on Human Rights (especially Articles 2 and 14).

17 For a discussion of other features of this sort of discrimination, see my 'What is the good of health care' in *Bioethics* 1996; **10** (October): 269–92.

18 Here again I rely on arguments first articulated in my 'Ethical issues in geriatric medicine' in Tallis R, Fillet H and Brocklehurst JC (eds) *Textbook of geriatric medicine and gerontology*, 5th edn (London: Churchill Livingstone, 1998, in press).

19 Does the proscription on killing include animals and plants? Are some commandments more important than others? Is the prohibition against coveting neighbours' oxen as (or more) important as that against coveting neighbours' wives?

20 See, for example, Ronald Dworkin *Taking rights seriously* (London: Duckworth, 1977, Chapter 5) and his *A matter of principle* (Cambridge, Mass: Harvard University Press, 1985, especially Part Two); and also his *Freedom's law* (Oxford: Oxford University Press, 1996, especially Section II).

21 This does not of course purport to be a complete account of either morality or moral reasoning.

22 Here I use the term 'hard case' in a way different to but consistent with Ronald Dworkin's famous discussion of hard cases in his *Taking rights seriously* (London: Duckworth, 1977, Chapter 4) and in *A matter of principle* (Cambridge, Mass: Harvard University Press, 1985, Chapter 5).

23 The judgements of the House of Lords in the Tony Bland case made clear that those in persistent vegetative state are also in a different category. See *Airedale NHS Trust* v. *Bland,* [1993] 1 All ER 858 (H.L.) and my 'Euthanasia and the value of life' in John Keown (ed) *Euthanasia examined: ethical clinical and legal perspectives* (Cambridge: Cambridge University Press, 1995: 6–22, 36–45 and 56–61). For those (including the author of this paper) who take a 'personhood' view, a view which locates the specially important moral claims and entitlements that we associate with 'human rights' not in human beings but in creatures with personhood, these anomalies are more easily reconciled. See John Harris *The value of life* (London: Routledge and Kegan Paul, 1985, Chapter 1).

24 See my 'The rationing debate: maximising the health of the whole community. The case against: what the principal objective of the NHS should *really* be' in *British Medical Journal* 1997; **314**: 669–72.

8 | Ageing in developing countries

Alexandre Kalache
Chief, Ageing and Health Programme, World Health Organization, Geneva

Ingrid Keller
Programme Assistant, Ageing and Health Programme, World Health Organization, Geneva

This chapter addresses the rapidity of the ageing process in the developing countries, the interrelated demographic, epidemiological and socio-cultural factors, and its public health implications. This is followed by a description of the model of 'healthy ageing' with a life-course perspective, which incorporates the need for appropriate policies within a conceptual framework of health promotion and the strengthening of primary health care.

The fast ageing process in the developing world

One of the main achievements in the 20th century has been a considerable increase in the numbers and proportions of older people in both developed and developing countries. Throughout the world populations are ageing. Today, there are around 540 million elderly people (60 years of age or over) living in the world with an estimated 330 million of them in developing countries. By the year 2025 there will be over 1,000 million people aged 60 years or over worldwide. As shown in Table 1, of the eleven countries with the largest elderly populations, eight will be in the developing world, namely China (284 million), India (146), Brazil (32), Indonesia (31), Pakistan (18), Mexico (17), Bangladesh (17) and Nigeria (16 million).

From 1990 to 2025 the rate of increase in the number of older people is expected to be up to 10 times higher in developing countries such as Colombia, Malaysia, Kenya or Thailand than in European countries. These developing countries are expected to experience a greater than 300% increase in their elderly

Table 1. Changes in the population of countries that will have more than 15 million people aged 60 and over in 2025

	Rank in 1950	Population aged over 60			Rank in 2025
		1950	2000	2025	
China	1	42.5	134.5	284.1	1
India	2	31.9	65.6	146.2	2
USSR	4	16.2	54.3	71.3	3
United States	3	18.5	40.1	67.3	4
Japan	8	6.4	26.4	33.1	5
Brazil	16	2.1	13.9	31.8	6
Indonesia	10	3.8	14.9	31.2	7
Pakistan	11	3.3	6.9	18.1	8
Mexico	25	1.3	6.6	17.5	9
Bangladesh	14	2.6	6.5	16.8	10
Nigeria	27	1.3	6.3	16	11

Source: Kalache[12]

populations over a period of only 35 years. Figure 1 shows the rapid ageing process – the increases in the total population of adults, particularly those aged 60 and over, will exceed those for younger age groups.

The demographic transition

From a demographic point of view, population ageing is characterised by a decrease in mortality as well as declining fertility. In other words, more people reach old age while fewer children are born. Over the last fifty years mortality rates in developing countries have declined – dramatically raising the global life expectancy at birth from around 45 years in the early 1950s to about 64 in 1990. This figure is projected to reach 73 years by 2020.[1] Furthermore, there are more than 20 developing countries today in which the life expectancy at birth is already above 72 years, for example Costa Rica, Argentina, Malaysia and the Republic of Korea. Table 2 shows the total fertility rates (defined as the average number of children a woman is expected to have at the end of her reproductive period) and the life expectancy at birth for selected countries. The differentials between developing and developed countries for total fertility rates – ranging from 6.9 for

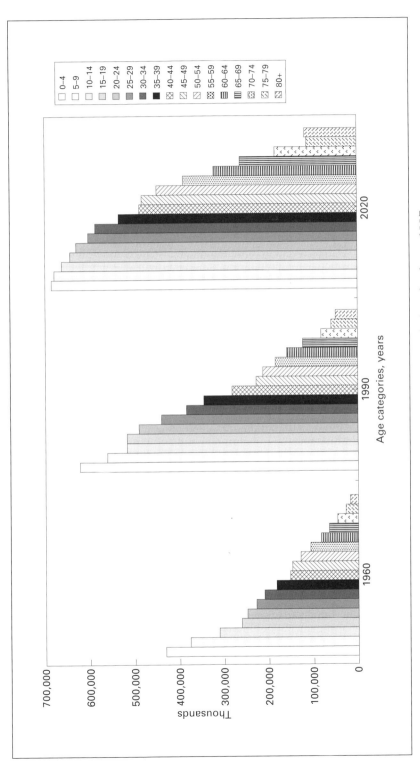

Fig 1. *Global population, age structured – changes over time.* Source: UN population database, 1997

Table 2. Total fertility rate and life expectancy at birth in selected countries – changes between 1960 and 2020

| | Total fertility rate | | | | Life expectancy at birth | | | |
	1960	1980	2000	2020	1960	1980	2000	2020
India	5.8	4.8	3.3	2.1	45	55	65	72
China	5.9	2.3	1.8	1.8	49	68	74	77
Brazil	6.2	3.8	2.7	2.2	56	64	68	73
Nigeria	6.9	6.9	5.8	3.0	40	49	56	65
United States	3.3	1.8	1.9	1.9	70	75	78	80

Nigeria to 3.3 for the United States in 1960 – as well as for life expectancy – ranging from 40 years to 70 years for the same countries in 1960 – will have been greatly reduced by the year 2020.[1]

Underlying causes for the demographic transition in what are the developed countries of today were mostly related to the gradually improving living standards of the majority of the population over a relatively long period following the industrial revolution. Improved housing conditions, sanitation and personal hygiene along with safer and better foods contributed to the slow but gradual decrease in mortality and fertility rates. Technological breakthroughs in the field of medicine were much later contributions to this process. In Norway, for example, it took about 100 years for the mortality rates to halve (1825–1925), while the same occurred in Brazil within about 30 years in the middle of this century.[2] This example shows that in the developing countries the growth of the aged population has been much faster. It is most likely accounted for by medical interventions based on the use of advanced technology and drugs, which are effective in treating and preventing diseases that kill people prematurely. Such interventions often anticipate economic development. The ultimate consequence is that today's poor adults and yesterday's undernourished children will become tomorrow's aged: a very different process than the one in today's industrial countries. Declining fertility rates can also be attributed to the use of modern, effective contraceptive means, often being part of campaigns especially targeted at women.

The epidemiological transition

Despite the substantial decrease of communicable diseases in

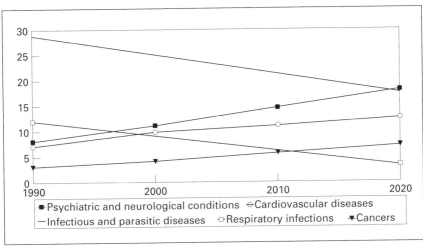

Fig 2. *Changes in non-communicable and communicable diseases in India between 1990 and 2020 (as % of total DALYs).* Source: WHO 1996[3]

developing countries (still serious threats to public health), non-communicable diseases are increasingly becoming prominent. It is projected that non-communicable diseases will account for 77% of all deaths in developing countries by the year 2020 (50% in 1990), while communicable diseases, which accounted for 41% of all deaths in 1990, will drop to 12%.[3]

Figure 2 illustrates this phenomenon for India.[3] While infectious and parasitic diseases are expected to experience a sharp decline in the coming decades, mental illness as well as cardiovascular diseases will increasingly account for years of healthy life lost (expressed in DALYs, ie disability adjusted life years; this measure 'is the sum of years of healthy life lost either through premature death or as a result of life lived with a disability'[4]). Furthermore, population ageing is expected to magnify the extension of mental health problems over the next quarter century. For instance, the number of people affected by senile dementia in Africa, Asia and Latin America is estimated at 22 million today and may exceed 80 million by 2025.[5] This is largely a reflection of the increased life expectancy for people with mental disorders and the rise in global life expectancies. Another example is the rise of visual impairments and vision loss related to increasing age, particularly of senile cataract. In most countries of Asia and Africa, it accounts for more than 50% of all blindness and more than 40% of all 'low vision' cases.[5]

The resulting 'double burden' (persisting communicable diseases and expanding non-communicable diseases) is a great challenge for public health authorities. Policies to be developed will have to pay close attention to costs. When searching for solutions, financial aspects have to be taken into account. For instance, in 1994 Japan's gross national product (GNP) per capita was US$34,630 and that of the United States US$25,880. Current GNPs for countries such as Indonesia (US$880), China (US$530), Pakistan (US$430) or India (US$320)[6] show that even if un-precedented economic development occurs, uninterruptedly for the next few decades, resources will be limited. Even the richest countries are now having difficulties in adapting to the new demographic order. Therefore it is vital for the developing countries not to adopt the highly medical and technologically advanced solutions embraced by the industrial countries: they will be unaffordable. Innovative, cost-effective interventions and models of good practice are urgently required.

Social and cultural changes affecting aged people

The impact of urbanization

Rapid urbanization has been a major trend over the last two decades and it is expected to be a persistent demographic feature for the foreseeable future. Figure 3 shows this for some countries with the largest population worldwide. For instance, it can be seen that the percentage of urban population is expected to double in China, Bangladesh and Indonesia between 1990 and 2020. Urbanization is largely due to the migration of the young from rural areas to the cities. Elderly relatives are left behind often looking after dependent (grand)children.[7] The responsibility for nourishment and education of the dependent (grand)children leads to physical strains on the aged, themselves often suffering from disabilities and health problems succeeding a life with poor nutrition and heavy physical demands. In Zimbabwe, for example, 35% of the rural elderly lived in skip-generation households, ie grandparents and grandchildren, in the mid-1980s, suggesting that the middle generation has migrated into the cities, seeking employment. Additionally, the increasing AIDS pandemic, heavily affecting today's middle generation, especially in Sub-Saharan Africa, is aggravating the problems. In urban households, on the other hand, aged persons are more likely to live in conjugal or two-generation (with unmarried children) households.[8] Those older persons who follow their children into the city face a life in alien environments, without social bonding to neighbours and friends, depending on

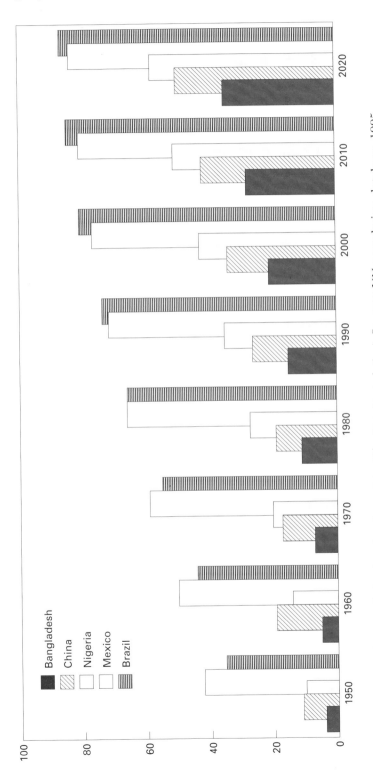

Fig 3. *Increase in urban population in selected countries (% of total population).* Source: UN population database, 1995

their children's meagre incomes. Trends towards a split family or the nuclear family also reflect a decline of traditional values. So far, customary values and financial constraints seem to be outstanding reasons why the proportion of elderly people living in institutions remains very low in developing countries. In the mid-1980s the proportion of people aged 65 and over living in institutions was 0.1% in Iran, 0.7% in Botswana and 1.5% in Brazil, as compared with 3.5% and 7.5% in Switzerland and Japan, respectively.[9] However, the pressures towards institutionalisation are already being felt throughout the developing world.

Women – today's carers and tomorrow's?

The increasing share of women in the paid labour force is also eroding traditional forms of care. As shown in Table 3, considerable increases in the number of women in the paid workforce has taken place in several developing countries. Since women, the traditional carers of aged family members, are now opting more and more for extra-household occupation, other ways have to be found for delivering care to the disabled old – or even more importantly to extend health expectancy.

Table 3. Women's share of adult labour force (age 15 and over)

	1970	1990
High human development		
United Arab Emirates	4	12
Costa Rica	18	28
Mexico	19	30
Chile	22	30
Uruguay	26	39
Republic of Korea	32	39
Medium human development		
Cuba	20	36
El Salvador	21	32
Brazil	24	34
Sri Lanka	25	34
Indonesia	30	39

Source: UNDP[6]

Social security and pension schemes

In the absence of comprehensive social security systems, most developing countries cannot provide pensions or other forms of financial support to their aged populations. In part this is due to the fact that a high proportion of people work in the informal sector, thereby not sustaining social security schemes. Some pension schemes, as is the case in Brazil for example, are unfairly generous for the well off.[10] Prolonged participation in the paid labour force or dependence on the income of children are the resulting consequences for most elderly. In Argentina, for example, 24% of men aged 65 or over and 4% of women in the same age group are employed; respective figures for Liberia are 70% for men and 33% for women. In comparison, in Austria only 2% of men and 1% of women in the same age group were permanently employed in the mid-1980s.[11] Alternative systems for supporting older populations in developing countries are urgently required.

Healthy ageing for a fulfilling old age

Keeping in mind the above discussed financial and socio-cultural constraints discussed above, medically advanced, highly specialised geriatric care will not be affordable for most aged people in the near future. Living longer offers unprecedented opportunities for fulfilling personal and social lives, but it also presents individual and societal challenges related to quality of life in old age. Therefore the WHO Ageing and Health Programme has adopted a life-course perspective to promote health throughout the life cycle, aiming to prevent functional and mental decline for as long as possible – adding life to years not only years to life. Older persons should be actively contributing to society for as long as possible. This does not necessarily mean inclusion in the formal paid work-force. In this agenda it is often difficult to 'quantify' the contributions brought by elderly people to society – as carers and promoters of societal cohesion.

A combined approach to health promotion in old age includes the improvement of the physical and the social environment as well as the provision of acceptable standards for health services. In terms of functional capacity this means to achieving the highest possible fitness level in early adulthood supported by health-promoting interventions such as physical activity (which is a powerful preventive measure for cardiovascular diseases, osteoporosis and back pain) or an adequate diet (a calcium-rich diet can help to prevent osteoporosis in women many years later). The decline of functional capacity can be delayed through similar prevention strategies, always expressed into culturally and ethically appropriate terms and adapted to individual situations. For individuals who have fallen below a disability threshold, cost-effective interventions to restore function (eg cataract surgery) or an increase in quality of life are aimed at. Here traditional forms of caring and healing, community-based approaches – without relying solely on the family, ie daughters or daughters-in-law – and well trained primary health care personnel are needed. Restructuring of the curricula is urgently needed, especially in terms of training, which has in the past been focused on maternal and child care.

Action for healthy ageing

The Ageing and Health Programme aims at taking the global lead to promote healthy and active ageing – it is never too late to promote health. The Programme's key components include database strengthening, advocacy, community-based programmes, research, training and policy development. The 'Brasilia Declaration on Ageing' – the outcome of two consecutive workshops in 1996 – was launched in summer 1996 as a first step in policy development. In summer 1997 a research initiative on healthy ageing in developing countries was prepared, aiming to identify the determinants of healthy ageing as well as assessment methodologies. The goal is to provide packages to countries that want to approach the development of ageing policies in a systematic manner.

References

1   United Nations. Population database. 1995.
2   Ramos L, Perracini M, Kalache A. *Journal of Cross-Cultural Gerontology* 1993; **8**: 313–23.
3   WHO. *Investing in health research and development*. Report of the Ad Hoc Committee on Health Research Relating to Future Intervention Options. Geneva, 1996.
4   WHO. *World health report*. Geneva, 1997.
5   WHO. *Population ageing: a public health challenge*, Fact Sheet No. 135. Geneva, 1997.
6   United Nations Development Programme. *Human development report*. New York: Oxford University Press, 1997.
7   Kalache A. Future prospects for geriatric medicine in developing countries. In: Tallis R, Fillit H, Brocklehurst J (eds). *Textbook of geriatric medicine and gerontology*, 5th edn. 1998, in press.

8   Hashimoto A. Urbanization and changes in living arrangements of the elderly. In: *Ageing and urbanization.* New York: United Nations, 1991.

9   United Nations. *Demographic yearbook,* Special issue: household and family structure. New York: UN, 1989.

10 Inactive workers, inactive congress. *Economist* 1997; June 7: 60–2.

11 Kinsella K, Taeuber C. *An aging world II,* International Population Reports P95/92-3. Washington DC, US Department of Commerce, Bureau of the Census, 1993.

12 Kalache A. Ageing in developing countries. In: Pathy MSJ (ed). *Principles and practice of geriatric medicine,* 2nd edn. Chichester: Wiley, 1991: 1517–27.

9 | Intergenerational equity: the politics and economics of an ageing population

Malcolm L Johnson
Professor of Health and Social Policy, University of Bristol

Our immortality resides in what we leave behind to influence future generations. If some part of us, as individual beings, continues to live in lives beyond our own we have achieved one dimension of immortality. The motivation to leave such a mark is central to the human condition and to all cultures and societies. So when Groucho Marx famously said 'Why should I care about posterity? What's posterity ever done for me?', he encapsulated one of the most enduring philosophical debates. The contract between the generations is a notion as old as history and one reformulated in every age. Today the twin forces of demographic change and the bundle of changes in outlook gathered under the term 'post-modernity' demand fresh thinking. Both the nature of social solidarity and what it means for people in later life have to be re-thought.

The intergenerational contract

Wherever people live in society, they do so in relationships of differing kinds which bind them both within and across generations. Whether these relationships are properly labelled family or kinship systems is a technical issue. But what universally characterises them is a set of rules or laws, guidelines and conventions which set patterns of obligation involving different degrees of reciprocity.

The nature of this solidarity between individuals and within the fabric of organised society has been articulated in recent centuries by Hobbes, Locke and Rousseau, through Bentham and Mill to the contemporary writings of Rawls, McIntyre and others. The common ground between these thinkers is their concern to link consent with obligation as integral features of civil society. Philosophers and political scientists recognise this stream of social

analysis as contractarianism – an acknowledged bond between
people who are both kin and strangers to each other and to their
children's children.

As Peter Laslett points out in his book with James Fishkin, *Justice
between age groups and generations*,[1] there are profound difficulties in
articulating the contractual nature of intergenerational exchanges;
which in turn are magnified by attempts to consider the 'processual' nature of justice over time. This is the essential conceptual
element in the discourse about an intergenerational compact and
the consequent issues of equity, which lie at the heart of this
chapter. There are, of course, practical concerns about the willingness and capacity of governments and economic systems to deliver
the resources to support elderly populations. These are more
questions of political conviction than of economic possibility, in
advanced societies. What will unlock the political uncertainty,
based as it is on short-term strategies and misconceptions about
the 'burdens' of an ageing population, is a newly refurbished
notion of generational solidarity.

As Harry Moody[2] points out, the character of generational giving
and receiving is transitive. 'We "repay" the generosity of the preceding generation by giving in turn to our successors'. Indeed this
apparent paradox is virtually universal. It is, to repeat Laslett's
term, processual. But even if life can be metaphorically depicted as
a procession, it is also one which stops at points in the life path to
engage in a series of ritual exchanges. Following nurture to adulthood there may be a period of dependent 'apprenticeship' –
college or low earnings early in a career – and a parental transfer
to enable the establishment of an independent household, perhaps
through marriage.

The appearance of grandchildren may prompt further gifts as
might financial misfortune or ill health.[3] But as the journey leads
the older generation to their last years, the often unspoken
dialogue of emotional support and services in kind in the un-
specified expectation of inheritance is acted out. Empirical
evidence of this is to be found in long-term care where relatives
seek to restrict expenditure to minimise diminution of their
inheritance.[4]

Impact of an ageing population

So what has changed to bring these theoretical issues into the
central area of debate about the young and the old? It is, of course,
the spectacularly beneficial reduction in this century of premature

death, which has led to what we now choose to call an ageing population. In turn it gives rise to the question – can we afford to support so many old people?

For the first fifteen years of my time as a gerontologist, our struggle with politicians and policy-makers was to get them to acknowledge the inevitability of the demographic explosion. But politicians rarely think more than three years ahead. So they listened politely and did nothing of any significance. The more forward thinking were genuinely exercised by the scale of the issues raised and tried hard to place the new old age on the agenda. More money and skilled person power was put into health and social services. Special housing assumed greater prominence. In America the gathered might of the 30 million members of the American Association of Retired Persons along with the feisty interventions of Maggie Kuhn and her Gray Panthers created what Henry Pratt called 'the Gray Lobby'.[5] In Europe older people's organisations have had less impact, not least because they presented no electoral threat. But unfortunately, about the time when recognition of a permanently changed world population structure dawned on those who make public policy, the world economy went into decline.

In the uncertainty about how to behave, two kinds of reaction emerged, one operational and the other rhetorical. The rhetoric declared a continuing commitment to older people, but one which had to be managed down because the financial and caring burden would be unmanageably great. Unrefined extrapolations of steeply rising pensions, housing, health and social care costs produced by actuaries and statisticians fuelled a sense of political panic.

Observing the consequences for national exchequers and therefore for taxation levels, a new vocabulary of individual responsibility grew in resonance with political shifts to the right. Within a remarkably short time it became one kind of received political wisdom that making your own provisions for health care costs and for income in later life was a freedom.

In practice it meant two things – privatisation of public services and cost-cutting. To bolster the logic we were told that the collectivism of state welfare initiative is costly, inefficient and has failed. In its place we needed free market disciplines, entrepreneurship and the cost efficiency which results from competition.

It was not only the pressure from a developing global capital market, wanting tighter control of national budget deficits, which militated against the variety of welfare states in Europe. As Esping-Andersen's penetrating analysis revealed,[6] the social class, labour market and public–private balance had so markedly changed in the post-World War II period that existing welfare regimes had less popular support both from those who had paid for them – the growing middle class – and from those who were the recipients of non-employment benefits. He argues persuasively that the growing middle class (which resulted from increased education and changes towards a post-industrial economy) was well disposed to the market model. Their disposable income was potentially increased and they were provided with more choice in ensuring the well-being of their own families.

The combination of class shifts, greater and more successful participation by women in paid employment and the success of a layer of ethnic minority people in education and work-based income are important elements in the dilemmas I want to address. It is too simplistic to suggest, as some commentators have, that the threat to retired populations is market economics.

We shall return to these other variables and the role they play. Nonetheless the rapid impact of New Right thinking on services and income for the old was substantial. Restraints have been placed on state pension levels; encouragements to join private pensions schemes have massively expanded the personal financial services sector; and direct services have been both outsourced and reduced.

What began as a localised infection became an international epidemic. Demographically induced gerontophobia began to manifest itself on an inter-continental scale. In most of the countries in Europe 50% or more of hospital beds were occupied by elderly people in addition to the 5–9% of the retired population resident in long-stay accommodation. To address the need to reduce expenditure, community care policies were introduced. The twin benefits of care at home where older people preferred to be, along with a presumed cost-effectiveness, drove a policy which few countries resisted. A late entrant, Canada, in its statement *Future directions in continuing care*[7] expressed the policy thrust with great clarity.

> ... community based care should be the service of first option where appropriate: public and professional attitudes consistent with this should be fostered ... . Continuing care should be to supplement or support, not replace, family and community caregiving.

Then the economic imperative follows:

> Continuing care services should be developed to support the lowest cost alternative appropriate to the needs of the individual.

In case the reader feels that in Europe we could not adopt such economic rationing for care, the excellent European Commission Observatory Report[8] provides the corrective. The report draws attention to the commonality of European policy concerns. It suggests there are five main issues:

- To contain the heavy growth of health expenditure.
- To define policy priorities for the rapidly growing group of elderly persons.
- To provide adequate coverage for the growing need for long-term care.
- To reorganise long-term care.
- To introduce new incentives for the development of community care and informal care.

Overall, community-based services across Europe have grown over the past decade, particularly in Denmark, Greece and Germany. But in Belgium the policy of blocked budgets has seen provision reduced. In Britain the number of home helps fell 30% between 1976 and 1988. Similarly in the Irish Republic the reduction in long-stay beds was not matched by the expansion of community care. The report from Italy stresses that about 15% of elderly people need home care but only about 1% receive it. A further spasm of cost-cutting has followed across the board cuts in a whole range of public services and social security benefits in New Zealand. Remarkably the example provided by a country with a population the size of Madrid, which managed its affairs so badly it was virtually bankrupt, became a model to be admired and reproduced by previously mature nations. Such a willingness to implement untested, unevaluated policies because of their potential to reduce the call on the middle class taxpayer should disturb us all as citizens as well as in our role of gerontologists.

These twists and turns in public policy bring me to summarise the main areas of cost reduction and draw out of them a selection of dilemmas they represent for all our societies. We can see in the literature a series of shifts in the principal life domains of family; work; health; well-being and housing; and income. To take the last first, we have seen concerted attempts to curtail and reduce expenditure on social security payments and pensions. It must be acknowledged that in this century there have been significant improvements in the financial position of retired people. But researchers still report unacceptable levels of old age poverty. The Netherlands has low levels of official poverty with 17% below the poverty line. But in Portugal and Spain, Perista[9] estimates the proportion is over 50%; in

Britain Walker[8] estimates 28%; whilst pensioners in France and Germany can be described in Alber's words as 'living in relative affluence rather than in relative poverty'.[10]

Whether we place the reaction within the overtly inter-generational contest represented by the middle-aged, middle class American pressure group, Americans for Generational Equity, or adopt Esping-Andersen's class/structural arguments, we can recognise a hiatus in the willingness to improve further the financial lot of older people. This, combined with the marked shift away from state to private pension, suggests it is possible to observe a reformulation of the bond between generations which we will further inspect shortly.

Into post-modern retirement

My analysis so far has raised many issues both for the political economy agenda and for public policy. But on this occasion I wish to focus on just one central issue which has ramifications for all of the others – retirement.

Retirement from regular paid employment can be traced back to the middle of the 19th century when civil servants were eligible to retire on a small pension. It was not until later in the century when Bismarck introduced a national system in Germany that the currently recognisable system began to appear. Bismarck chose the age of 70 because by that stage most workers were genuinely old and unable or becoming unable to work. Today the average expectation of life at birth in northern Europe is about 75 years for men and about 80 years for women. A hundred years ago it was more than 15 years less and fewer than 4% of the population lived beyond age 65 (today 15% of the population is aged over 65 – and that figure will reach 18% (20% in some countries) by about 2020).

Retirement was originally designed only for employed men, in selected occupations and with minimal financial support. Moreover, it was both the expectation and the reality that the vast majority lived for only a short time and in poor health. Most workers carried out manual tasks in unhygienic and unsafe work places; so that over a work life of 50 years they become progressively more sick. Those who survived to 65 were likely to be exhausted. Young and Schuller[11] put it graphically in their book *Life after work* when they say:

> Retirement was a kind of postscript to work which only had to be defined negatively. The watch or clock that employers traditionally handed over to their retiring workers was a deceit. It symbolised the

gift of the time that was now to be their own rather than the employers! But the new owner was going to wear out long before the watch.

Until recent times, therefore, almost everyone worked either until they died or until they were physically incapable of continuing to work on. Life after work was only for a few survivors and for them it was an ante-chamber to death.

When the Old Age Pensions Act was introduced in Britain in 1908, the age of 65 was adopted – as it was in most countries of Europe, though a few delayed until age 70. Again it applied only to selected occupations and only to men. In the inter-war years the retirement concept extended across the developed world eventually embracing all occupations and including women.

The post-World War II era of welfare states exemplified by those in Scandinavia and Britain made retirement and adequate state pensions available to almost everyone. Yet in this early postwar period elderly women were still seen in black clothing, virtually excluded from social life and treated as invalids. Indeed retirement, old age and dependency became virtually synonymous both in the public mind and in public policy.

As an evangelist for the full citizenship of old people, I am now acutely aware that the contemporary patterns of retirement – beneficial as they are – are unsustainable in their present forms. More to the point, the life of extended leisure presently experienced by growing numbers of retirees is not what was ever meant in earlier conceptions of intergenerational support to the old. Such a contract must rest upon a principled reinterpretation of what is equitable and what is deliverable.

I have no doubt whatever that rich nations like our own can more than adequately provide for all its citizens of all ages. It will have to open closed and buttressed doors such as those of the immensely wealthy pension funds and re-examine inheritance practices, to release more of our collective assets. But we can – and will – sustain the whole population without damaging the well-being of the young and middle-aged. The essential elements of the present system of basic state pensions and largely free health care can be funded so long as there is a constraining realism about the limits of the rights and the responsibilities which are integral to the contract.

In health care we will be forced into more sensible, but socially sanctioned, rationing on the basis of the probability of real health gain and to doctors sharing the treatment functions with other health practitioners.

As for retirement as we have come to know it over the past two decades – it will have to be radically reassessed. Society cannot afford to forgo the direct contribution of so large a segment of its adult population. Between two and three decades of living outside of the mainstream of economic life is a breach of the contract. The commitment younger generations have made is to support those who cannot support themselves, not to provide an ever growing sabbatical in the third age. By the same token, third age people will not tolerate exclusion from full citizenship. Nor will many of them be willing or able to exist economically on fixed and diminishing incomes (think what your salary was 20 years ago).

The capacity to continue to earn income will become an imperative for many young old, both for current living and for the avoidance of a penurious late life. So in rethinking the generational contract it is essential that there is a reliable platform of services and pension provision for all. But the post-60 phase of life will need to be much more flexible:

- Flexible retirement between 55 and 75 may need to be considered.
- New opportunities for job changes in mid and late career – possibly to lower paying jobs, but ones which can go on much later, eg in the service sectors of industry and in the expanding realms of social and health care – should be available.
- The care of the old old is increasing the responsibility of the over 55s. Mechanisms need to be found to include some of this in the formal economy.
- New generations must – like in earlier times – make provision for their own old age a lifetime investment. I say this knowing all too well that there are structural inequalities which will make this difficult or impossible for some. It is properly within the social contract for just and non-stigmatising provision to be made for them.

Time does not allow me to develop this argument about the reconstruction of later life and its links with generational justice. However, I hope enough has been said to persuade you that I continue to reject the panic which characterises global political thinking; but accept that older people must resume some of the responsibility to society from which postwar retirement policies have released them.

My arguments are not political in construction but ethical. If the post-modernist malaise is not to overtake developed societies, they must make positive attempts to renew the social solidarity which still holds us together. We, and our children, must be willing to look beyond our Saga holidays and cultural pursuits for the sake of a greater social good. The preservation of the intergenerational contract is vital to human societies in the new millennium. As ever it will require reciprocity. Universal retirement as we know it will have to go.

References

1   Laslett P, Fishkin J. *Justice between age groups and generations.* New Haven: Yale University Press, 1992.

2   Moody HR. *Ethics in an aging society.* Baltimore: Johns Hopkins University Press, 1992.

3   Daniels N. *Am I my parents' keeper? An essay on justice between the young and the old.* Oxford: Oxford University Press, 1988.

4   Crystal S. *America's old age crisis.* New York: Basic Books, 1982.

5   Pratt HJ. *The politics of old age.* Chicago: University of Chicago Press, 1976.

6   Esping-Andersen AG. *The three worlds of welfare capitalism.* Cambridge: Policy Press, 1990.

7   Health and Welfare Canada. *Future directions in continuing care.* Report of the Federal/Provincial/Territorial Sub-Committee on Continuing Care. Ottawa: Health Services and Promotion Branch, 1992.

8   Walker A, Alber J, Guillemard AM (eds). *Older people in Europe: social and economic policies.* Report of the European Observatory. Brussels: Commission of the European Communities, DG V, 1993.

9   Perista H. *Social and economic policies and older people in Portugal.* Lisbon: GEGIS, 1992.

10 Alber J. Health and social services. In: Walker A, Alber J, Guillemard AM (eds). *Older people in Europe: social and economic policies.* Report of the European Observatory. Brussels: Commission of the European Communities, DG V, 1993.

11 Young M, Schuller T. *Life after work: the arrival of the ageless society.* London: Harper Collins, 1991.

10 | Medicine and old age: the research agenda

Shah Ebrahim

Professor of Clinical Epidemiology, Royal Free Hospital School of Medicine, London

Setting research priorities is a topical game which everyone wants to play. The prize for the investigator is continued employment, for the administrator control of resources, and for the politician the delight of being seen to do something. Different players have set out their stalls, defining how they see research in old age for the future (Table 1). The lack of coherence between these different research priority lists is striking: it must be assumed that there is only limited agreement about what should be done. Furthermore, the composition of the groups convened to examine research priorities has an impact on the final list of topic areas.

Does this matter? Since resources for research in old age are very limited it may be of particular importance that the 'right sort of research' gets funded. However, the large-scale research that has been funded on ageing in the UK does not appear to have been driven by priority setting exercises.

The Medical Research Council[1] has put major resources into trials to examine efficacy (screening the over 75s, treatment of hypertension), observational studies of cognitive function and ageing, incontinence services, and has set up AGE-NET, a collaborative network of investigators. Both the scope and volume of activity are at odds with the priority list. Using priorities to make policy which can then be operationalised and implemented as research programmes appears to be much more difficult than simply drawing up the lists.

By contrast, the Department of Health[2] has assumed that all policy initiatives have the capacity to tackle the issues of ageing and longevity, and consequently has no central priority list but does have a huge amount of research activity funded by the National Research and Development programme relevant to old age listed in its National Research Register. The projects are generally small

Table 1. Research priorities for medicine in old age

Medical Research Council	World Bank	NHS Executive (North Thames)
Population projections	Drug trials in poorer countries	Rehabilitation services
Health status measurement	Elder abuse and neglect	Mental health services
Use of health services	Hospitalisation trends	Palliative care services
Inequalities	Inequalities	Health/social care interface
Efficacy of interventions	Counselling and selfhelp	User involvement in planning
Rehabilitation	Traditional healers	Health promotion
Organisation of care	Causes of cardiovascular disease	Efficacy of interventions

Sources: Medical Research Council[1]
World Bank: Consultation on the Health of the Elderly. 1993 World Development Report. London School of Hygiene & Tropical Medicine, 1992
NHS Executive (North Thames): Health of Older People R&D Programme, Commissioning Document, November 1996, NHS Executive North Thames, London

scale, lacking power to detect clinically important effects, and concern efficacy (but seldom costs) of interventions and thus give no useful information for option appraisal.

Worryingly, the research questions are formulated in a reductionist way (eg 'In diabetic patients is a practice nurse able to provide effective and safe foot care?') but such information will be difficult to synthesise into practical approaches to defining how the health *system* might be improved (eg what is the optimal balance of work for a practice nurse?). Consequently it is unlikely that this body of work will fulfil the needs of the National Health Service for information that will be influential, definitive and widely applicable.

The medical research charities have a major place in defining priorities through how they choose to fund research. In the main, the research is disease orientated (eg Stroke Association, British Heart Foundation, Alzheimer's Disease Association), with the exception of Research into Ageing which has taken a strong biological approach rather than a social, population or health services approach.

What research is the right research?

It might be argued that any research in a Cinderella area like ageing is better than no research. Simply doing research to know more is a valid objective, but may not be a good enough reason to persuade the public to find the cash. The Commission on Research for Development[3] have considered the role of research, defining four main purposes: (1) to identify and set priorities among health problems; (2) to guide and accelerate application of knowledge to solve health problems; (3) to develop new tools and fresh strategies; and (4) to advance basic understanding and the frontiers of knowledge.

Without such a framework for developing a research agenda, it seems likely that essential links in the research system (Fig 1) will be lost and public support for a science-based approach to development will wane.

Barriers to research

Ageing and the consequences of longevity are complex phenomena which touch on biology, sociology, epidemiology, demography, economics, welfare, environment, architecture and design, leisure and social facilities, to name a few. A uni-disciplinary

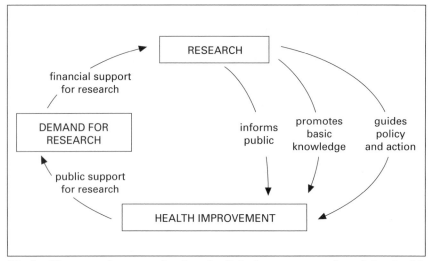

Fig 1. *The research system showing the links between research activity, health improvement and demand for research.* Source: Commission on Research for Development[3] (Reproduced with permission)

approach is unlikely to yield the insights needed to provide fresh strategies to solve existing or future problems. In Britain, our national research councils are a heritage of past ways of thinking and working – more appropriate for the 19th century than the 21st. Ageing, more than most topic areas, highlights the intellectual poverty of single discipline approaches to defining questions and answering them.

Moving to trans-disciplinary research is not easy as it requires a more integrated training of scientists, larger research groups, willingness to collaborate, and a vision that is broad enough to accept that no one discipline has all the answers.

My own research agenda attempts to approach the questions surrounding longevity from the following perspectives:

- what are the causes of increased life expectancy?
- what are the effects of increased life expectancy?

The causes of increased life expectancy

Genetics (see also Chapter 11, by Kirkwood)

Perhaps the most tantalising question surrounding ageing is the oldest question: why do we age? The search for elixirs of youth, or more recently the genes that regulate ageing phenomena, is of understandable interest. Genetic research offers the promise of prediction of longevity and of modifying the effects of genes that adversely affect survival and predispose to age-associated diseases. The fruits of the massive investment in molecular genetics are beginning to be seen in the areas of diagnosis and treatment for a small number of conditions. Obviously, the question of why we age is of little relevance to the question of why life expectancy changes and the implications of such changes. It does not seem likely that genetic research will provide the means of altering the rate of age-ing of individuals sufficiently to have an impact on population life expectancy, which is affected by much more powerful social, economic, environmental and personal factors.

Life expectancy

The most striking aspect of ageing over the last century has been the rapid increases in life expectancy experienced by many populations all over the world, even in poorer regions.[4] A fundamental question is why are we living so much longer? More specifically, the differential life expectancy of different populations is of considerable interest. Table 2 shows trends in life expectancy at 65 years of age and at birth in different parts of Europe. What is striking is the difference between the Central/Eastern European countries and the more economically advantaged European Community countries. Men in Central and Eastern European countries

Table 2. Life expectancy at age 65 years and at birth in different parts of Europe, 1974–91

Region/Country	Change in life expectancy 1974–91, at age 65 (years)		Change in life expectancy 1974–91, at birth (years)	
	Male	Female	Male	Female
Central/Eastern	−0.1	0.4	−0.3	1.5
Nordic	1.2	1.7	2.5	2.5
United Kingdom	2.0	1.8	4.2	3.4
European Community	1.9	2.4	3.7	4.1
Portugal	1.9	2.7	4.6	5.5

Source: World Health Organization, Health for All dataset, Copenhagen regional office

have experienced a fall in their life expectancy at age 65, suggesting a worsening of mortality rates from common killers in old age – heart attacks and strokes. Perhaps even more surprising are the gains made by Portugal, which remains one of the poorest countries in Europe. However, absolute levels of poverty do not correlate strongly with life expectancy in Europe; income disparities appear to be more important, but only partial, predictors of life expectancy.[5]

Explaining why life expectancy differs between places – why do the Japanese live so long? – has been an interesting puzzle for some time.[6] Possible factors include environmental and personal risk factors for common diseases, economic and social development, health and social policy, and interactions between these factors. Untangling such complex variables is difficult because of problems of measurement, lack of relevant data, and the fact that when things are improving, any factor that is also changing will show a correlation, an ecological fallacy. The new and adverse situations facing people in Central and Eastern Europe provide novel research opportunities. Ecological trend analyses will be more powerful as the factors of likely causal relevance will be those that are associated with improvements in life expectancy in Western Europe and with deteriorations in Central and Eastern Europe. In addition, cohort studies making measurements of individual risk factors and linking these with subsequent disease will be required to provide stronger evidence of causality. Hypotheses that merit attention are that variation in life expectancy is due to quality of medical care, environmental pollution, socioeconomic factors and health behaviours (eg diet, smoking, alcohol, stress).[7]

Healthy active life expectancy (HALE)

If we accept that the purpose of health and social policy in older age is to extend the length and quality of life, an understanding of the determinants of life expectancy is of fundamental importance to developing preventive health and social policy. However, understanding the causes of *healthy active life expectancy*[8] is of greater importance but is much less easy to study because of a lack of relevant data. Interestingly, although the Medical Research Council defined research into HALE as of major importance,[1] no relevant work has been commissioned or funded.

Studying the determinants of HALE requires a series of nationally representative cohort studies to be established measuring both the onset of relevant disabilities and also mortality.[4] Such study designs – *cohort sequential studies* – are relatively rare, partly because of the long-term leadership and organisational commitment required and also because cohort studies have an undeserved reputation of being expensive. The cohort sequential design provides transitional probabilities of becoming disabled (and also of recovery) at different ages and, most importantly, allows an assessment of whether these probabilities are getting better or worse among successive cohorts of older people.

Establishing and maintaining such studies requires an adequate infrastructure of epidemiologists, statisticians, social scientists and demographers with interests in ageing. While such research groups exist, achieving long-term funding of a sufficient scale to recruit and follow up cohorts of around 10,000 people has not been feasible in the UK. An approximate cost of £100,000 per annum per cohort is required based on experience with single cohort studies in cardiovascular disease. This failure of funding agencies is disappointing given the UK's pre-eminence in health services for elderly people and the calibre of its social scientists, epidemiologists and demographers.

An alternative option to the cohort sequential design is to conduct periodic national disability surveys.[9] These have the advantage of being easy to set up and interpret but run the risk of falling out of the priority list of funding bodies as they may not appear interesting enough. The major scientific disadvantages of cross-sectional studies are that recovery from disabled states is discounted and no allowance is made for cohort effects. What this means in practice is that effects of interventions that might alleviate disability would be missed, and disability rates of today's 75-year-olds have to be applied to 75-year-olds in the future, which may lead to over-estimation of disability projections.

The lack of commitment by the previous government to collection of information to evaluate health and social policy is shown by their decision (attributed to the Office for National Statistics) to cancel the 1997 national General Household Survey (GHS). The serial nature of this survey is vital for trend analysis and it provides the only source of disability measurements over time in England and Wales.[8] It is to be hoped that the GHS will be restored by 1998 as it is relatively inexpensive – £500,000 – but gives us the basic information on trends to evaluate policy at a macro-level.

Fortunately, the Department of Social Security has agreed to fund a further national disability survey which should provide comparable data to the earlier study[9] and provide a picture of how disability rates have changed over the last decade.

The effects of increased life expectancy

The spectre of an ageing society with increased levels of dependency, inability to afford the pension bill, and social collapse is frequently presented. The up-beat World Bank vision[10] of how to avert the old age crisis and make money through ill-researched and unstable private sector pension schemes is also questionable. It is vital that we have relevant data to examine the consequences of increased life expectancy and thus avoid potentially damaging stereotypes of elderly people as an intolerable burden on society or a windfall money-making opportunity.

Reversible disability

Disability rates rise almost exponentially with age and by the age of 80 years four out of five people have some self-reported disability.[9] Evaluation of the reversibility of this disability is of considerable importance. Some of it will be 'hard-core' and extremely difficult to deal with, whereas other disabilities may be easy to reverse in the early stages but become more intractable if detected and managed late in their natural history. A possible framework for defining a research agenda is shown in Fig 2.

Figure 2 emphasises the need for a trans-disciplinary approach to reducing and reversing disability. Single discipline research can provide solutions to disability but may miss the benefits of lateral or alternative approaches. For example, a trial of occupational therapy provision of aids in the bathroom demonstrated a clear benefit,[11] but missed those patients who might have benefited from a diagnosis of a reversible proximal myopathy, or replacement of a worn out hip joint.

Currently, we have little information on the contributions of disease, the environment and the individual to the experience of disability, and even less idea of the relative costs and effects of intervening in each of these areas. For example, what are the relative merits (eg in terms of acceptability, or social engagement) of increasing social welfare allowances for loco-motor disabled people compared with improving the built environment, or provision of more day centre facilities? In an ideal – or perhaps resource rich – world we would do all these things; in reality we have to make choices. What choices do we make when we have no information to guide us on costs and benefits?

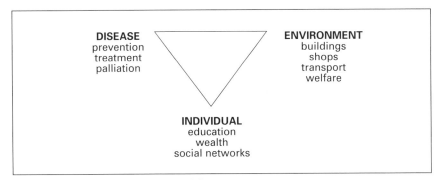

Fig 2. *The causes of reversible disability*

Cost-effectiveness of health and social care

Evaluation of the cost-effectiveness of interventions used for elderly people forms a large part of the existing Health Technology Assessment programme of the Department of Health's Research and Development programme. Since elderly people are the greatest consumers of health care, small changes in what is spent may bring disproportionate gains or expenses. It is necessary to focus attention on those conditions that contribute most to HALE as this is where the greatest gains from new knowledge will occur. Figure 3

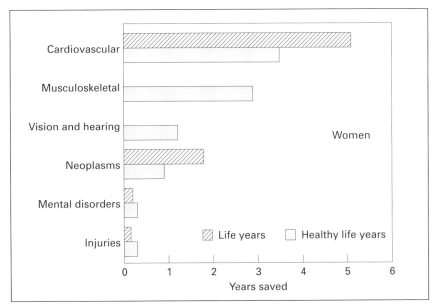

Fig 3. *Life years and healthy life years saved by the elimination of specific diseases.* Source: Bone *et al*[8]

shows the savings in life expectancy and HALE that would arise if disease groups were eliminated. Obviously, this is not a realistic possibility but it does provide a reasonable way of determining priorities for research.

Prevention. The clear priorities for research are cardiovascular diseases, locomotor problems – chiefly osteoarthritis, vision and hearing impairments, and depression. In cardiovascular disease much is known about aetiology but much less is known about effective means of behaviour change or the relative costs and effects of fiscal versus lifestyle interventions. In osteoarthritis and depression more knowledge is needed about modifiable risk factors which will enable preventive strategies to be developed. However, it could be argued that if the main objective is to increase HALE, rather than life expectancy, the best way to do this would be to focus on those areas that contribute more to HALE but less to life expectancy.

Trials. It is essential that more elderly people are included in randomised controlled trials of new (and old) drugs for common diseases as they are the main consumers of many drugs. Achieving this may require specialists in care of elderly people to be more actively engaged in the design and organisation of clinical trials. This will require training which should be built into the 'research' part of specialist registrar training.

In addition to drug trials, evaluation of models of care (eg home versus hospital; nurse-led versus consultant-led) and of specific rehabilitation methods (eg Bobath stroke physiotherapy versus physical fitness approaches) are needed. There are major difficulties in carrying out trials of complex interventions such as rehabilitation. Many of the problems are methodological: devising an appropriate placebo; blinding of participants and evaluators; defining the intervention; ethical issues; fixed beliefs of efficacy of rehabilitation. Obtaining sufficient funds for conducting large-scale trials which involve a major health service intervention is extremely difficult. Trials requiring therapists or nurses to provide interventions such as rehabilitation or counselling are expensive and it is becoming clear that the NHS is generally unwilling or unable to find the money for such interventions even when research bodies are able to fund the evaluation costs.

A further problem is that of the research cultures of different health professions involved in complex interventions. Doctors are well-versed in the merits of randomised controlled trials whereas nurses and therapists are more experienced in single case and observational study designs, often using qualitative methods of data collection, which are relatively weak methods of evaluating the efficacy of specific interventions. Progress is being made in the area of stroke research, largely through the efforts of the Stroke Association and the British Stroke Research Group, which have encouraged the formation of multidisciplinary research groups and have promoted the randomised controlled trial but have not denigrated alternative methods of enquiry. More emphasis on scientific method is required in the training of all health professions at undergraduate and postgraduate levels.

Long-term care, both in the community and in institutions, is of considerable importance because of the misery associated with low quality care, the large numbers of people requiring such services, their high cost, and the limited evidence of effectiveness of different options (eg social versus nursing models of care). The Departments of Health and Social Security have commissioned several research projects in the institutional care area which aim to determine the characteristics of 'good' nursing homes and the cost-effectiveness of case management. Far more work is required on the economics of long-term care, interventions to support carers, and the wider use of community rehabilitation and palliative care among long-term care patients.

Social and economic consequences

A major concern about increased life expectancy is the effect on tax burdens required to provide adequate social and health care. Demographic research aimed at making more accurate projections of the elderly population, broken down by disability, social and economic status, will be essential for forecasting future needs. Of particular interest is the impact of personal long-term care insurance and the shift of burdens from the state to individuals. Inter-generational support or conflict are possible consequences of increased life expectancy: more information on those factors that promote support and reduce conflicts would be helpful in formulating policy. For example, involving older people in schools as co-teachers in verbal history projects has been very successful, as has using schools as lunch clubs for older people. Evaluation and extension of such work would be of great value in improving the quality of both younger and older people's lives.

In summary, research priorities for life expectancy fall into two broad areas: understanding its *causes* and its *effects*. Research into life expectancy, and more importantly, healthy active life expectancy requires new, large-scale, national cohort studies to be established and maintained. Such data will allow monitoring of the success (or failure) of health and social policies on ageing. The concept of *reversible disability* is helpful in defining a trans-disciplinary research agenda focusing on disease, the environment and the individual. Evaluation of the cost-effectiveness of specific interventions, particularly complex non-pharmacological treatments, requires much greater investment in both methodology and health service commitment. Finally, the economic and social consequences of increased life expectancy also deserve research, and fundamental to this are better projections of changes in population structure, together with social research directed at the aims, aspirations and needs of the population in caring for frail, very elderly people.

References

1   Medical Research Council. *The health of the UK's elderly people.* London: MRC, 1994.
2   Department of Health. *Research for health.* London: Department of Health, 1993.
3   Commission on Research for Development. *Health Research. Essential link to equity in development.* New York: Oxford University Press, 1990.
4   Ebrahim S, Kalache A. *Epidemiology in old age.* London: BMJ/WHO Publications, 1996.
5   Power C. Health and social inequality in Europe. *British Medical Journal* 1994; **308**: 1153–6.
6   Marmot MG, Davey Smith G. Why are the Japanese living longer? *British Medical Journal* 1989; **299**: 1547–51.
7   Bobak M, Marmot M. East–West mortality divide and its potential explanations: proposed research agenda. *British Medical Journal* 1996; **312**: 421-5.
8   Bone M, Bebbington A, Jagger C, Morgan K, Nicolaas G. *Health expectancy and its uses.* London: HMSO, 1995.
9   Martin J, Meltzer H, Elliot D. *The prevalence of disability among adults. OPCS surveys of disability in Great Britain*, Report 1. London: HMSO, 1988.
10 World Bank. *Averting the old age crisis. Policies to protect the old and promote growth.* London: Oxford University Press, 1994.
11 Hart D, Bowling A, Ellis M, Silman A. Locomotor disability in very elderly people: value of a programme for screening and provision of aids for daily living. *British Medical Journal* 1990; **301**: 216–20.

11 | Genetics and the future of human longevity
*F E Williams Lecture**

Thomas B L Kirkwood
Professor of Biological Gerontology, University of Manchester

The first half of the 20th century saw a rapid increase in expectation of life in industrialised nations due to improved sanitation, public health, housing, nutrition and medical skills. The second half of the 20th century has seen a growing concern with the biomedical challenge generated by the increasing prevalence of old people in society. Much of this work has focused on genetics. It is perhaps noteworthy that the discovery by Watson and Crick[1] of the double helical structure of DNA occurred in the same decade as the first formal theories on the evolution of ageing were proposed by Medawar[2] and Williams,[3] and when two mechanistic theories of ageing, the free radical and somatic mutation theories, were suggested by Harman[4] and Szilard,[5] respectively. A union of evolutionary and mechanistic theories occurred in 1977, in the form of the disposable soma theory of ageing.[6,7] In recent years the evidence for genetic factors being involved in ageing has expanded at a great rate.[8-10]

The major lines of empirical evidence for the role of genetic factors in ageing are as follows: first, lifespan in human populations shows significant, though low, heritability[11,12] (in the order of 20–35%); second, different species have different intrinsic lifespans which can reasonably be attributed to differences in their genomes; third, in human populations there exist inherited progeroid disorders such as Werner's syndrome[13] in which affected individuals have a complex phenotype characterised by premature development of a variety of age-related diseases, including arteriosclerosis, type II diabetes, cataracts, osteoporosis and cancers; fourth, in invertebrate model systems such as the fruit fly, *Drosophila melanogaster*, and nematode worm, *Caenorhabditis elegans*, clear evidence of genetic effects on lifespan has been discovered.[14,15]

*This lecture was first published in *J R Coll Physicians Lond* 1997; **31**:669–73.

As the 20th century draws to its close, the amount of genetic information concerning human health and disease is expanding at an enormous rate, due to the efforts of the various human genome projects. What will be the impact of research on human longevity in the 21st century and beyond? It is already clear that the science of human ageing will be perhaps the pre-eminent biomedical research challenge in this period.

Terminology

In human gerontology the words 'ageing' and 'senescence' are used more or less interchangeably, and this will be the practice here. This is not to deny the importance of development and maturation, which some also count as 'ageing', but my primary concern is with the declines in structure and function that unfold gradually and progressively during adulthood. The measure of senescence most commonly used is one based on the increase in age-specific death rates.[16,17]

Gompertz[18] observed that human mortality rates show an approximately exponential rise with increasing chronological age, and similar patterns have been noted in other species.[17] The Gompertz model has been generalised by adding a constant to represent age-independent mortality due to extrinsic causes,[19] and the resulting model for mortality rate can be written as:

$$u(x) = \alpha e^{\beta x} + \gamma$$

where α, β and γ are constants and x denotes age. The parameter β denotes the 'actuarial ageing rate' and determines how fast the age-dependent component of adult mortality increases with time. The parameter α denotes 'initial vulnerability' and acts as a scale parameter for the age-dependent component of adult mortality (note that the Gompertz model does not make any attempt to describe juvenile mortality). The parameter γ denotes the age-independent component of adult mortality. There is some evidence that human mortality increases more slowly among centenarians[20] but it is not yet clear whether this slowing at extreme old age reflects: (i) genetic heterogeneity within the population, (ii) particularly assiduous care of the oldest old, or (iii) intrinsic biological processes. Genetic heterogeneity is likely to be at least part of the explanation as centenarians probably comprise a genetically robust subset of the population with slower rates of biological ageing than the rest.[11]

An exponential increase in mortality rates within human populations does not require that the underlying physiological processes follow exponential kinetics. Cross-sectional studies reveal great variability in both the slopes and patterns of the changes observed with age. However, many important diseases of late life do show exponential increases in age-specific incidence; examples include Alzheimer's disease, carcinoma of the prostate and carcinoma of the colon.

Theories of evolution of ageing

Theories of evolution of ageing seek to explain why ageing occurs and to identify what kinds of genes are responsible, how many of them there are likely to be, and how they might have been modulated by natural selection. The puzzle, of course, is to explain why ageing occurs in spite of its clearly deleterious impact on Darwinian fitness.

Because ageing is so obviously deleterious for the individual, attempts have been made to explain its evolution in terms of an advantage to the population as a whole.[21] Is it a form of population control to prevent overcrowding? This theory is given little credence today – first, because there is no evidence that animal numbers in the wild are regulated to any significant extent by senescence, most deaths occurring at younger ages from extrinsic causes such as predation, and second, because they invoke group selection, which is unlikely to be effective in this context. Nevertheless, these ideas periodically reappear, presumably because they appeal to the notion that ageing is programmed like development and will yield to the same kinds of genetic analysis that has proved so successful in developmental biology.

Greatest weight is now attached to evolutionary theories which are 'non-adaptive', in the sense that they do not suggest ageing confers any fitness benefit *of itself*, and they recognise that it may indeed be harmful. The non-adaptive theories explain evolution of ageing through the *indirect* action of natural selection.

One such theory is the 'mutation accumulation' theory.[2] This is based on the observation that natural selection is relatively powerless to act on genes which express their effects late in the lifespan at ages when, because of *extrinsic* mortality, survivorship has fallen to a low level. The assumption is that in the starting population there would be no age-related increase in intrinsic mortality, otherwise the theory would be circular. In such a context, late-acting deleterious mutations are predicted to accumulate over a large number of generations within the genome. The practical consequences of such an accumulation would be minimal in the wild environment but will have a serious effect upon the organism if it is moved to a protected environment. In the protected environment, the reduction in extrinsic mortality permits survival to ages when the intrinsic effects of the accumulated mutations are felt. In other words, ageing has evolved.

A second concept invokes the idea that there may be pleiotropic genes whose expression involves trade-offs between early-life fitness benefits and late-life fitness disadvantages.[3] Like the mutation accumulation theory, this 'antagonistic pleiotropy' theory rests on the observation that the declining force of natural selection provides a differential weighting across the lifespan which will ensure that quite modest early-life fitness benefits outweigh major fitness disadvantages in later life.

The trade-off principle is also at the heart of the 'disposable soma' theory.[6,7,22] This theory provides a direct connection between evolutionary and physiological aspects of ageing by recognising the importance of the allocation of metabolic resources between activities of growth, somatic maintenance and reproduction. Increasing maintenance promotes the survival and longevity of the organism but only at the expense of significant metabolic investments that could otherwise be used for greater reproductive effort. It can be demonstrated with formal models that the optimum allocation strategy results in a smaller investment in maintenance of the soma than would be required for indefinite lifespan.[23,24]

Three categories of genes are thus predicted by the evolutionary theories to affect ageing and longevity:

1. Genes for somatic maintenance and repair, as well as the gene regulatory elements that control the settings of these genes.
2. Pleiotropic genes involved in trade-offs that do not include somatic maintenance.
3. Purely deleterious late-acting mutations that have escaped elimination due to the decline in the force of natural selection at old ages.

Martin *et al.*[10] have suggested the terminology 'public' and 'private' to distinguish genes associated with ageing that are likely to be shared or individual. Genes involved in trade-offs, especially genes regulating fundamental aspects of somatic maintenance such as antioxidant systems, are expected to be public. Conversely, late-acting deleterious mutations are expected to be private, since the fate of these alleles will be strongly influenced by random genetic drift.

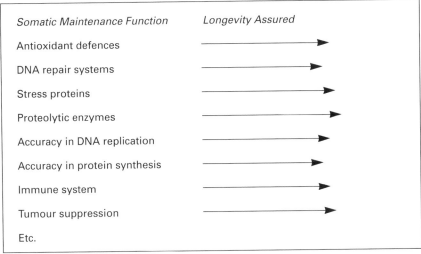

Fig 1. *Diagram illustrating how polygenic control of longevity is effected, as predicted by the disposable soma theory of ageing.* Natural selection acts in a similar way on the different genes regulating individual somatic maintenance functions. The precise setting of each function in an individual determines the period of 'longevity assured', as indicated by the lengths of the arrows. At the level of the population, the average period of longevity assured by each maintenance function is expected to be similar. However, some variance within the population is expected, so that within and between individuals the relative lengths of the arrows may vary. (Adapted from reference 7)

Implications of the evolutionary theories

Several implications follow from the evolutionary theories. First, it is predicted that multiple kinds of genes contribute to senescence and that the total number of such genes may be large (Fig 1). This suggests that uncovering the genetic basis of senescence will be a complex task requiring a combination of approaches, such as quantitative trait locus mapping, adaptation of methodologies for analysis of polygenic diseases, transgenic animal models, and so on.

Second, the theories readily explain differences in the rate of ageing between different species, which are likely to be the result of different levels of extrinsic mortality. This is because extrinsic mortality determines the rate of decline in the force of natural selection. Extrinsic mortality also has a major effect on the optimal allocation of energy between maintenance, growth and reproduction. The disposable soma theory predicts higher levels of maintenance in somatic cells of long-lived species, for which there is growing evidence.

Third, in the case of the disposable soma theory, there is a clear prediction that the actual mechanisms of senescence will be stochastic, involving processes like the random accumulation of somatic mutations or oxidative damage to macromolecules. Biological gerontology has long been divided between the'programme' and 'stochastic' views. The idea that ageing might be due to the accumulation of random damage, but that the *rates* of damage are programmed in a statistical sense through the evolved settings of the maintenance systems, offers some accommodation of these apparently opposite views.

A fourth implication of the evolutionary theories is that senescence may be malleable, through modification of the factors that affect decline in the force of natural selection and through alteration of the balance between good effects and bad that are implicit in the theories that invoke trade-offs. Indeed, from the human perspective, the trade-off principle is one that needs to be borne in mind when considering possible interventions in the ageing process. Interventions that would increase longevity or postpone a late-age disease may turn out to have side effects due to the existence of trade-offs.

Genetics of human longevity

Two strategies have been delineated to identify genes associated with human longevity.[11] The major interest is in genes that may confer above-average or extreme longevity, since there is potentially a large number of alleles that shorten lifespan through mechanisms that are unconnected or only indirectly connected with ageing.

One strategy is the 'candidate gene' approach using case-control methodology. The aim is to identify extremely long-lived individuals and compare their allele frequencies at the candidate gene locus to the allele frequencies of a control population, who will be less long-lived individuals from the same genetic background. This assumes that the controls are unlikely themselves to reach the extreme old age of the 'cases', which is not unreasonable if the age criteria are appropriately defined. Candidate gene studies have identified significant differences in allele frequencies between centenarians and controls at the HLA,[25,26] apolipoprotein E[27] and angiotensin converting enzyme loci,[27] but these have not so far been applied to their full potential.

The second approach is the sib-pair method designed to detect loci that segregate within kin groups with traits of interest, such as inherited diseases. In the case of ageing, the trait of interest is extreme longevity. This method requires the recruitment of a sufficiently large sample of extremely long-lived sib pairs and its application has not yet been reported.

In the case of progeroid diseases, 1996 saw the identification by positional cloning of the gene responsible for Werner's syndrome which appears to code for a DNA helicase.[28] This finding is highly significant in that it supports the idea that accumulation of DNA damage may be a contributing factor to ageing, especially in dividing cells. In patients with Werner's syndrome post-mitotic tissue is relatively spared, which is consistent with the discovery that the gene defect is one that will principally affect DNA replication.

The future of human longevity

Our present understanding of the genetics of human ageing permits some consideration of how human lifespans might conceivably change in the future, although a great deal more research will be needed. Human longevity may be altered as a result of (i) natural selection, (ii) artificial selection, (iii) genetic engineering, (iv) drug interventions, (v) genetic risk assessment coupled with prophylactic measures, (vi) behavioural and lifestyle modifications.

Natural selection

Even though human populations now live in circumstances that many regard as 'unnatural', the process of Darwinian natural selection continues. The fact that so many humans now live to experience old age will, in principle, expose the genetic factors involved in ageing to new selection forces tending to increase lifespan. On the other hand, selection against inherited weaknesses has been diminished through medical interventions and the generally more comfortable circumstances of life, and this may lead to the accumulation of minor gene defects that will eventually have deleterious effects on long-term survival. Patterns of reproduction have also altered profoundly through the development of reliable contraception, resulting in extensive family planning governed mostly by social and economic circumstances. The net effect of these changes on the genetics of the future human life history are hard to predict but merit consideration.

Artificial selection

Artificial selection has produced significant effects on the life histories of fruit flies,[29,30] but such procedures are neither ethical nor feasible in human populations. The fruit fly experiments are interesting for the information that they provide on genetic variance in populations and on the rate and extent of the response to selection. However, the genetic variance within a population reflects the evolutionary history of that population, and there are likely to be major differences between fruit flies and humans with regard to the genetic variance in factors affecting lifespan.

Genetic engineering

In the popular mind, advances in genetic research are often linked to the idea of genetic engineering. Genetic engineering is a conceivable route to modification of human longevity although this presupposes major advances in the technology of gene therapy and in the detailed dissection of the genetic factors influencing lifespan. At present, effective gene therapy is still unavailable even for monogenic inherited diseases such as cystic fibrosis which are, rightly, the primary targets of research. Whether genetic modification of a 'normal' process like ageing will ever be ethically acceptable or practically feasible is far from clear, and meaningful discussion must await the further identification of possible genetic targets. Nevertheless, the broad issues can and should be addressed as part of the wider debate on application of the 'new genetics'.

Drug interventions

Drug interventions based on understanding of genetic mechanisms involved in late-life diseases such as Alzheimer's disease, are the most likely immediate benefits to emerge from genetic advances in ageing research. Whether these will, in time, have the cumulative effect of altering underlying lifespans remains to be seen, but in any case the more urgent and attainable goal is to improve the quality of the later years of life.

Genetic risk assessment

One of the major successes of genome research to date has been the identification of risk alleles for conditions such as Alzheimer's disease and breast cancer. The discovery of alleles linked to late-life diseases is likely to continue at an accelerating pace. If such discoveries are coupled with the development of effective drug treatments or prophylaxis, they are likely to result in further extension of average life expectancy through reducing the negative impact of risk alleles on survivorship. It is less likely, however, that this approach will alter maximum lifespan, since the longest lived at present are probably those who are at lowest genetic risk.

Behavioural and lifestyle modifications

Advances in genetic understanding of ageing will not necessarily require genetic or drug-based interventions to produce enhancement in the quality of later life, or even life extension. Knowledge of genetic mechanisms is also likely to help to identify non-genetic factors (nutrition, exercise, etc) which may be beneficial. It is already clear that genes are only a part of what influences duration of life. The identification and exploitation of gene-environment and gene–lifestyle interactions will be of great importance too.

References

1 Watson JD, Crick FHC. Genetical implications of the structure of deoxyribonucleic acid. *Nature* 1953; **171**: 964–7.
2 Medawar PB. *An unsolved problem of biology.* London: HK Lewis, 1952.
3 Williams GC. Pleiotropy, natural selection and the evolution of senescence. *Evolution* 1957; **11**: 398–411.
4 Harman D. A theory based on free radical and radiation chemistry. *Journal of Gerontology* 1956; **11**: 298–300.
5 Szilard L. On the nature of the aging process. *Proceedings of the National Academy of Sciences USA* 1959; **45**: 35–45.
6 Kirkwood TBL. Evolution of ageing. *Nature* 1977; **270**: 301–4.
7 Kirkwood TBL, Franceschi C. Is ageing as complex as it would appear? New perspectives in ageing research. *Annals of the New York Academy of Sciences* 1992; **663**: 412–17.
8 Jazwinski SM. Longevity, genes, and aging. *Science* 1996; **273**: 54–9.
9 Kirkwood TBL. Human senescence. *BioEssays* 1996; **18**: 1009–16.
10 Martin GM, Austad SN, Johnson TE. Genetic analysis of ageing: role of oxidative damage and environmental stresses. *Nature Genetics* 1996; **13**: 25–34.
11 Schächter F, Cohen D, Kirkwood TBL. Prospects for the genetics of human longevity. *Human Genetics* 1993; **91**: 519–26.
12 McGue M, Vaupel JW, Holm N, Harvald B. Longevity is moderately heritable in a sample of Danish twins born 1870–1880. *Journal of Gerontology* 1993; **48**: B237–44.
13 Martin GM. Genetic syndromes in man with potential relevance to the pathobiology of aging. *Birth Defects* 1978; **14**: 5–39.
14 Tower J. Aging mechanisms in fruit flies. *BioEssays* 1996; **18**: 799–807.

15 Lithgow GJ. Invertebrate gerontology: the age mutations of *Caenorhabditis elegans. BioEssays* 1996; **18**: 809–15.

16 Kirkwood TBL. Comparative and evolutionary aspects of longevity. In: Finch CE, Schneider EL (eds). *Handbook of the biology of aging*, 2nd edn. New York: Van Nostrand Reinhold, 1985: 27–44.

17 Finch CE. *Longevity, senescence and the genome.* Chicago: Chicago University Press, 1990.

18 Gompertz B. On the nature and function expressive of the law of human mortality and on a new mode of determining life contingencies. *Philosophical Transactions of the Royal Society of London* 1825; **115**: 513–85.

19 Makeham WM. On the law of mortality and the construction of annuity tables. *Journal of the Institute of Actuaries* 1860; **6**: 301–10.

20 Smith DWE. The tails of survival curves. *BioEssays* 1994; **16**: 907–11.

21 Kirkwood TBL, Cremer T. Cytogerontology since 1881: a reappraisal of August Weismann and a review of modern progress. *Human Genetics* 1982; **60**:101–21.

22 Kirkwood TBL, Holliday R. Evolution of ageing and longevity. *Proceedings of the Royal Society of London B* 1979; **205**: 531–46.

23 Kirkwood TBL, Rose MR. Evolution of senescence: late survival sacrificed for reproduction. *Philosophical Transactions of the Royal Society of London B* 1991; **332**: 15–24.

24 Abrams PA, Ludwig D. Optimality theory, Gompertz' law and the disposable soma theory of senescence. *Evolution* 1995; **49**: 1055–66.

25 Proust J, Moulias R, Fumeron F, Bekkhoucha F, *et al.* HLA antigens and longevity. *Tissue Antigens* 1982; **19**: 168–73.

26 Takata H, Ishii T, Suzuki M, Sekiguchi S, Iri H. Influence of major histocompatibility complex region genes on human longevity among Okinawan-Japanese centenarians and nonagenarians. *Lancet* 1987; **ii**: 824–6.

27 Schächter F, Faure-Delanef L, Guénot F, Rouger H, *et al.* Genetic associations with human longevity at the *APOE* and *ACE* loci. *Nature Genetics* 1994; **6**: 29–32.

28 Yu C-E, Oshima J, Fu Y-H, Wijsman EM, *et al.* Positional cloning of the Werner's syndrome gene. *Science* 1996; **272**: 258–62.

29 Partridge L, Barton NH. Optimality, mutation and the evolution of ageing. *Nature* 1993; **362**: 305–11.

30 Zwaan BJ, Biljsma R, Hoekstra RF. Direct selection on life span in *Drosophila melanogaster. Evolution* 1995; **49**: 649–59.

12 | A correct compassion: the medical response to an ageing society
The Harveian Oration of 1997*

Professor Sir John Grimley Evans
Professor of Clinical Geratology, University of Oxford

In the words of one of his biographers, William Harvey was the first Englishman to be what we would now recognise as a scientist. 'He observed the facts as we observe them, he experimented as we experiment and he reasoned as we reason'.[1] In responding to the impact of the ageing of our population on medicine and society, we need to observe, experiment and reason. We also have to recognise that the responsibilities of the medical profession are now far wider and deeper than Harvey could have anticipated; medicine has become an institutionalised component of the social structure of the nation. As doctors, we accept the duty implied by Harvey to search out and apply the knowledge relevant to our craft. But the medical profession – as both a conscientious servant of the people, and a privileged elite – has a duty of concern for the policy as well as the practice of medicine. James Kirkup, in a poem honouring the surgeon Philip Allison, wrote of 'a correct compassion' whereby doctors translate their knowledge and human concern into practical and coolly appraised action.[2] Forty years later we are aware, sometimes uncomfortably, that a correct compassion has to extend beyond the patient in front of us to those who are not, or not yet, our patients but who may be affected by the decisions we make.

*The Harveian Oration is given annually at the Royal College of Physicians of London. The 1997 Oration was given on 15 October 1997, and is printed in full in a separate publication by the College; and also in *J R Coll Physicians Lond* 1997;**31**:674–84.

The ageing population

So far we have met only the first of two waves of ageing of the British population. At the beginning of this century Britain underwent the 'demographic transition' from a pattern of high birth and high mortality rates to one of low birth and low mortality rates common to all nations undergoing economic development. As national income rises there comes a point when, for reasons that are not always clear and probably differ between nations, infant and child mortality rates fall. There is then a lag, typically of a generation, before fertility and completed family sizes also decline. During this lag a bolus of unprecedented survivors of childhood is released into the population. This can be seen as a bulge in the population structure of England and Wales in the 1971 census (Fig 1). The passage of this cohort through old age has been largely responsible for the increase in numbers of older people over the past twenty years. The size of the elderly population will now become more stable for two or three decades. The new wave of population ageing will come with the arrival in old age of the cohort of post-war 'baby-boomers' in the third and fourth decades of the new millennium.

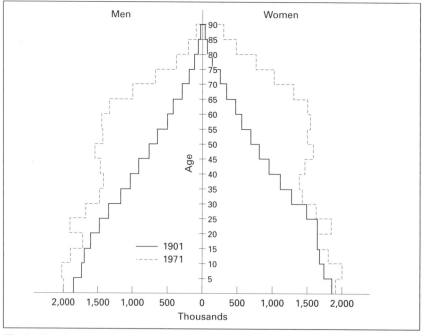

Fig 1. *Population pyramids of men and women in England and Wales: 1901 and 1971*

The second cause of ageing of populations, again linked to economic advancement, is a fall in mortality rates in middle age and later life. In the UK this has been continuous for women since the start of the century but in men the fall was delayed by the epidemic of coronary heart disease and smoking-related diseases. We do not know whether older people in the UK are living longer because they are fitter or because unfit and chronically ill people are being kept alive longer. These two processes, which may coexist, have very different implications for health and social services. One means of monitoring the needs for and the success of services for an ageing population would be by measuring some form of healthy active life expectancy (HALE) at later ages.[3,4] At present we have no adequate data on this in the UK. Suggestions that recent increases in total life expectancy in Britain involve prolongation of the average period of disability before death are derived from the General Household Survey (GHS).[5] The GHS estimates of disability are based on self-report only and its sampling frame does not include institutionalised people. It will register an increase in disability if improvements in community care enable more unwell older people to live in their own homes rather than having to move into institutions.

Where good data on active life expectancy are available an interesting paradox emerges. Table 1 presents data calculated from a study in Massachusetts over 20 years ago[6] but recent data from the Netherlands[7] show the same pattern. The partition of total life expectancy into dependent and non-dependent years shows that although women outlive men, their extra years are accounted for entirely by years of dependency. Moreover, women tend to marry men older than themselves and so are likely to bear their heavier burden of disability when widowed and in relative poverty. In the USA this pattern means that while only one in seven of men who

Table 1. Life expectancy in years; Massachusetts 1970–72. Calculated from Katz *et al*[6]

Age	Total		Active		Dependent*	
	Men	Women	Men	Women	Men	Women
65–69	13.1	19.5	9.3	10.6	3.8	8.9
70–74	11.9	15.9	8.2	8.0	3.7	7.9
75–79	9.6	13.2	6.5	7.1	3.1	6.1
80–84	8.2	9.8	4.8	4.8	3.4	5.0
85+	6.5	7.7	3.3	2.8	3.2	4.9

* Dependent: needing personal help with one or more activities of daily living

attain the age of 65 can expect to spend a year or more in a
nursing home before death, for women the figure is one in three.[8]

In the absence of clear indications of how age-associated
morbidity is changing, we can view the future only by projecting
current patterns of illness and disability, and use and costs of
services, onto future age structures. Figure 2 combines data on
disability[9] with population projections[10] to estimate the growth in
numbers of older people who will be affected over the next
decades. Many influences may intervene to mitigate the needs for
health care implicit in the figures. None the less, a correct
compassion requires us to prepare for the challenge they represent.

There are four things to be done: we must agree on what are to
be the aims of health care for an ageing population; we must
maximise the efficiency of the services we provide; we must
minimise the need for care by reducing the incidence of age-
associated disease and disability. First, however, we should think
about funding, for it would be probably unrealistic, and certainly
imprudent, not to expect costs of health and social services to rise if
ideologically and socially acceptable standards are to be sustained.

Funding

If patterns of practice and costs remain as at present the main
financial impact of ageing in the UK will fall on the long-term care

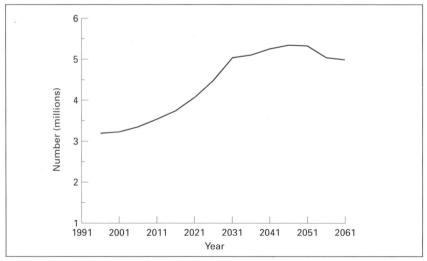

Fig 2. *Projected number of people in Great Britain with disability of grade 3 or
more (likely to require personal help).* Based on National Disability Survey[9] and
population projections[10]

sector rather than on acute secondary or primary care.[11] By the year 2030 expenditure on long-term care alone will amount to nearly 11% of the GNP, equivalent at present values to £2,000 per head of the population of working age, a rise approaching 50% on 1991 figures.[12] The dominance of long-term care in the predictions arises because at present the use of primary and secondary care rises much less steeply with age than does the use of the various forms of long-term care. We do not know if this pattern is clinically appropriate or economically efficient – it may partly be the product of accountancy rather than economics in apportioning costs between the health and the social service budgets. A fund-holding general practitioner may genuinely think it more efficient economically to save money in his budget by advising an old lady to go into a nursing home at the expense of the social services department rather than to have her painful hip joint replaced. The cumulative cost to the tax- and rate-payer, however, may be very much higher and the old lady much less happy. Advocates of age-based rationing of health services are too ready to assert that depriving old people of health care will necessarily save money.[13] Advances in technology are increasing the applicability of secondary health care to older and frailer people but policies aimed merely at capping costs may prevent full potential economic efficiency, as well as maximal clinical effectiveness to be attained.

Growth in health care should not be viewed in a purely negative light. There will be some savings from discontinuation of obsolescent forms of care although these are unlikely to be large. More importantly, growth in health care provides employment and is a stimulus to innovation. There is no evidence that the economy of the USA has suffered from the growth of its grotesquely inefficient system of health care.[14] Europe is ahead of the rest of the world in the ageing of its populations; this is an opportunity to be ahead in developing the appropriate technologies that the rest of the world will also come to need.

We have to identify the structure for future funding that carries highest social utility. This task is urgent. If an insurance model, private or social, is chosen this must be put in place soon if adequate funds are to accumulate by the time they are needed. We would also need to find interim arrangements to overcome the double burden that will hit the generation that is paying for its own future care by insurance and simultaneously for the care of others on the existing 'pay-as-you-go' model. At present the costs for long-term care of old people with resources are paid from the potential inheritance of their children, whether as fees or insurance premiums. This falls unevenly on families and is a source of guilt and unhappiness to old people, as well as raising other unpleasant possibilities at this time of glib chatter about euthanasia. An insurance philosophy calls for costs to be shared between those (but only those) who are at risk. An interim levy on inheritance would spread the costs among all potentially affected families.

A new element in debates about future funding of health care is that of inter-generational equity. It has been claimed, for example, that the generation of adults who introduced the welfare state will collect around four times as much from it as they put into it.[15] While that generation might claim that they deserved this for fighting or enduring the Second World War, the aged baby-boomers of the 2030s will, we hope, have no such claim on their successors. Although as an economic issue, inter-generational equity may have an unreal feel for many, it can have an important impact on social wellbeing in determining whether older people are seen as parasitic on the working population or merely receiving their agreed deserts. There is also a political dimension. The generation of baby-boomers who will generate the challenging expansion in health and social care costs in the 2030s are also the generation to bear the double burden of the overlap in transferring from pay-as-you-go to insurance funding. Their children who will pay the bills if the pay-as-you-go system is continued will not reach voting age and political potency until it is too late to fund an insurance model to underwrite the 2030s. Here is a prescription for political paralysis.

What are we trying to do?

The output of clinical health services comprises the changes induced in the wellbeing of individuals but there is a long-running ethical debate about how such health transitions should be valued. Old people in particular are caught in the tension between polar views of the aims of health services. The collectivist view is that outputs of health care should be valued on behalf of the State. This valuation will usually be in terms of some derivative of extra life-years obtained.[16] The individualist view is that a health change can only be valued by the person seeking or receiving it.[17] For the collectivist, increasing the wellbeing of old people generates little value because of their relatively short life expectancy and their economic unproductivity. The individualist view is that it is not permissible to value a person according to age or any other overt attribute. Whether an old woman values her remaining years of life more or less than a younger man values his will depend on individual circumstances and desires, not directly or predictably on sex, race, social class or age. Moreover, the comparison cannot validly be made; if the value of life lies in the subjective experience of being alive this is observable only by the person living the life. Individual valuations of lives cannot be brought under the scrutiny of a single observer and are therefore formally incommensurable. The notion that it is possible to overcome this incommensurability by the economists' device of willingness-to-pay analysis is illusory since this merely transfers the incommensurability problem from monadic valuations of living to monadic valuations of money. From this standpoint, piling life-years of different individuals together as if they were some aggregatable commodity like eggs from battery hens is intellectually as well as ethically indefensible.

Do we serve a collectivist or an individualist ideology? The answer may not be simple. A nation may espouse a mixed ideology as well as a mixed economy and circumstances may change. Collectivism is a necessity in war and may be the best response to poverty. We do not have a written constitution and can only seek the ideology of our nation in its history and in the common rhetoric of our political parties. English history since the traumas of the 17th century has been of a heterogenous people seeking peaceful and efficient ways of living together. My interpretation is that in times of peace, the fundamental values of society in the UK include respect for the uniqueness and sanctity of individuals, equality of citizens before the institutions of the State, and the right to live the lives we wish provided we respect the same rights of others. All our political parties preach freedom and, in the words of John Stuart Mill: 'The only freedom which deserves the name is that of pursuing our own good in our own way, so long as we do not attempt to deprive others of theirs or impede their efforts to obtain it'.[18]

To pursue this individualist ideal we must explore the measurement of health service outcomes in terms of the realisation of individually specified goals. This will be to sail against a strongly running collectivist tide. Evidence based medicine (EBM) is at present concerned with trials and overviews focusing on the average outcomes of treatments for diseases. This is valuable, but is sufficient only for the collectivist. The individualist doctor needs to treat patients, not diseases. Individualised evidence based medicine (IEBM) requires identification of individual determinants of outcome, and individualised objectives of care. Concealed in the average benefit of treatment in randomised mega-trials are patients who did not benefit or who were harmed. We need to know if those individual outcomes could be predicted. Given present

practical and statistical conceptions of mega-trials, relevant individual data are not collected or can be pursued only in post hoc sub-
group analyses, with the danger that the results will be treated as if
they were testing rather than generating hypotheses. Too often we
do not know how patients entering mega-trials were selected and
what population of patients they represent. This concern is
particularly relevant to old people who are more variable physiologically and psychologically than the young. Both for the pursuit
of IEBM and for assessment of cost-effectiveness, conventional
trials are the beginning, not the end, of evaluation of a treatment.

A second aim for IEBM is to embody individualised objectives of
care that reflect a patient's personal values and desires. An interesting development in this direction has been the extension of
personal construct psychology into health care.[19] Using an
interrogative technique built round the device of the repertory
grid it is possible to help a patient identify the dimensions of what
he or she regards as quality of life and to put values on each to
correspond to present and potential states after treatment.
Another empirical approach to the problem is exemplified in
interactive computerised programs to explore patient preferences
for the management of prostatic and menstrual problems.

Something of the particular importance of obtaining older
individuals' personal assessments of the value of interventions can
be seen in the discrepancies revealed in American comparisons of
what older people would want from health care compared with
what their potential proxies, family members or professional
advisers, think they would want.[20,21]

Whatever the outcome of the broader debate, there is common
ground for collectivists and individualists in the prevention of
disability which the individualist does not want people to have to
endure and the collectivist does not want to have to pay for. Most
older people fear disability and the dependency and loss of dignity
it brings more than they fear death. Disability is most usefully c-
onceptualised as arising from an ecological gap between what an
environment demands and what an individual is capable of doing.
At a clinical level this gap can be closed by therapeutic intervention to improve patients' capabilities and by prosthetic
measures to reduce the demands of their environments. At a
population level we should seek to make our environment less
disabling for an ageing population. Apart from issues of safer cities
and more rigorous traffic control, we can enhance the ease of
visual perception and cognitive mapping of outdoor and indoor
environments. As has repeatedly been said, and repeatedly ignored

by architects and planners, environments that are safer and pleasanter for older people are also safer and pleasanter for us all.

Efficiency of services

The importance of assessing the efficiency, in the sense of cost-utility, of services rather than merely the efficacy of treatments has been recognised in the growth of health services research (HSR) and health technology assessment (HTA) as major research domains. The UK developed its system of health care for older people pragmatically. Its underpinning lies in ready access of older people who fall ill to a full range of modern medicine informed by specialist geriatric expertise,[22] and embodying the four-stage 'process of geriatric care' summarised in Table 2. None of this has ever been adequately evaluated in the UK but studies of replications in the US have shown it to be more cost-effective than conventional care.[23] Whether this reflects the value of geriatric expertise or merely the poor quality of conventional care in the US is unclear, but American experience does give warning of the consequences if the British NHS were to lose the specialist vision and commitment of geriatric medicine.

For all its faults and lapses, the NHS has achieved wonders over its half century in providing effective, efficient and compassionate care for older people. We must doubt, however, if a successful future can lie merely in providing more of the past. A problem for

Table 2. The process of geriatric care

Assessment
     Health (diagnoses, prognosis)
     Function (physical, mental)
     Resources (culture, education, social, economic)
Agree objectives of care
     What does the patient want?
     What is feasible?
Specify the management plan
     To close the ecological gap between what the patient
     can do and what the environment requires:
          therapeutically – improve the patient
          prosthetically – reduce environmental demands
Regular review
     Is progress as expected?
     Does the plan need changing?

HSR for an ageing population lies in the difficulties in asking the strategically important questions. Innovation and research are restricted by rigid social and professional structures and political control at a time when we might do well to consider even the unthinkable. One radical example must suffice: British general practice enjoys favoured political status because it is seen as a throttle point for controlling costs. But we do not know in an evidence-based way that it is necessarily the most efficient means of providing primary health care. It is conceivable that in some situations, and for some groups of patients such as disabled older people with complex problems, primary health care might be better provided by specialist units as part of integrated primary and secondary care systems. We may never be allowed to find out by conventional means. A case for asking radical questions could be made from systematic and critical comparisons of health and social services in other nations, particularly in Europe. At present European research funds seem to be directed to semipolitical purposes concealed in concerted actions and pooling projects. These focus on our supposed or imposed similarities rather than on the more exciting scientific possibilities in exploiting the natural experiments of our differences, both in health and in health care.

Minimising the need for care

Disability in later life is rarely due to a single disease, and general age-associated processes are also contributory factors. For a strategic approach to reducing the need for services, we need to think about ageing as a whole and not just about specific age-associated diseases. Ageing in the sense of senescence is the loss of adaptability of an organism as time passes. Loss of adaptability at an organismic level is manifest in a rise with age in the risk of dying. In order to understand the evolution of ageing it is important to recognise that even if we did not age we would all still die eventually. Death would come from disease, accident, predation or warfare but the chance of death would be constant with age or might even fall as natural selection weeded out those less adept at staying alive. In the human species, senescence first becomes manifest around the age of 12 or 13 years when the age-specific mortality rates which fall from birth turn upwards. Then, after early perturbations due mostly to violent deaths, age specific mortality rises almost exponentially throughout adult life (Fig 3). Rates in men are higher at all ages than in women and as there is no discontinuity in the rates in later life, there does not seem to be any biological basis for distinguishing 'the elderly' from the rest of the human race. Death is a rather crude measure of loss of adaptability but the prevalence of disability also shows a continuous and exponential association with age.[9]

Loss of adaptability in ageing is caused by interactions between intrinsic (genetic) factors and extrinsic factors in environment and lifestyle. Extrinsic factors in ageing can be detected by conventional epidemiological methods, seeking differences in the ageing patterns of populations living in different places or different times. Extrinsic factors have been shown by such means to be relevant to age-associated trends in blood pressure,[24] hearing loss,[25] femoral fractures[26] as well as to the incidence of vascular disease and cancers. Figure 3 shows that the basic age pattern of total mortality rates in this country has not changed in the last 100 years although the level of mortality has fallen, particularly at young ages. The age of lowest mortality has not altered despite the enormous changes in environmental conditions and hazards over the last century (Fig 4). This suggests that it may be under intrinsic control; this is plausible given that evolutionary pressure would be expected to produce the maximum fitness of members of a species at the onset of reproductive capacity. It seems that maximum age at death has also not altered over the century. The problem here is that as more data are accumulated rarer events will be observed, which in turn

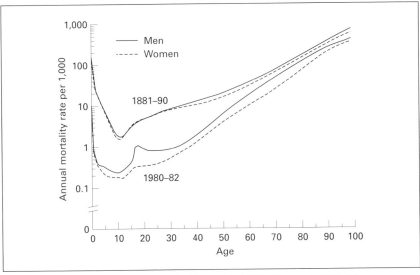

Fig 3. *Age-specific mortality rates in England: 1881–90 and 1980–82*

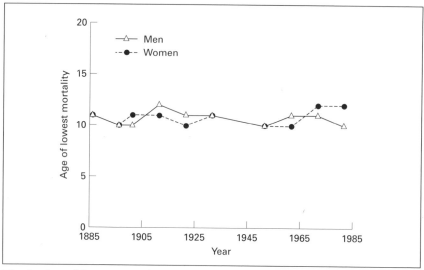

Fig 4. *Age of lowest mortality in men and women calculated from English life tables 1881–90 to 1981*

could give rise to an increase in maximum observed age at death even though the percentage of people reaching that age does not change. Figure 5 reveals an interesting feature of extreme old age. If life expectancy of women is plotted against age, it seems that life expectancy at late ages is asymptotic to zero but has not changed over time (Fig 5a). If the same data are plotted semi-logarithmically so that percentage rather than absolute differences are revealed, we find that the percentage increase in life expectancy at the age of 100 has been of the same order as that at younger adult ages (Fig 5b). The effects of extrinsic factors are apparent at age 100 but we cannot identify the age range over which they are active.

Identification of the period in life when extrinsic factors act is crucial in a search for interventions. Those citizens who will provide the challenge to the health services of 2030 are already among us and already in their thirties. Benefits from enhanced exercise levels, reducing blood pressure, and giving up smoking can be seen in middle age and later – for maximal benefit extrinsic factors may need to be controlled earlier in life. The amount of bone and muscle laid down in childhood and adolescence may be important determinants of disability in old age. Barker has pushed the origins of late age-associated vascular disease back into the uterine environment by linking measures of intrauterine development with hypertension and coronary heart disease in later life.[27] The

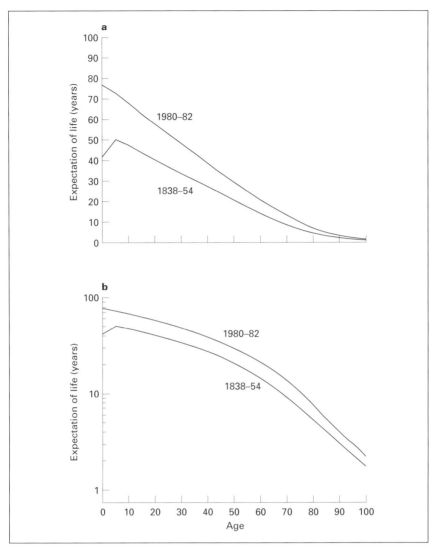

Fig 5. (a) *Simple plot of life expectancy of women in England: 1838–54 and 1980–82;* **(b)** *Semi-logarithmic plot of life expectancy of women in England: 1838–54 and 1980–82*

intrauterine environment can certainly do direct damage to a fetus as the fetal alcohol syndrome demonstrates, and subtler effects may emerge if the hypothesis of a uterine factor modulating the hereditability of intelligence survives further study.[28] Intelligence evolved because it improves survival; we must expect it to have a similar influence in modern society. Education as an enhancer of intelligence is potentially one of the most important extrinsic influences on the lifelong pattern of age-associated disease and disability.

If the Barker effect is confirmed, it may reflect the existence of a metabolic switch[29] allowing a fetus to adjust its metabolism to the sort of environment it is destined to be born into. Deprived fetuses could do well on average by switching on mechanisms for storing any excess energy as body fat, but to conserve resources in the longer term by restricting body size. If such a fetus finds itself in a better environment than foreshadowed it would be at risk of the metabolic consequences of relative over-nutrition. These consequences include a high risk of diabetes and vascular disease in middle life. The mechanism is analogous to that proposed for the possessors of the thrifty genes postulated in populations that have been under heavy selection pressure from famine,[30] and which may contribute to health problems of some immigrant groups in the UK[31]. If this is so we should not regard an infant from a deprived intrauterine environment as inevitably programmed to develop vascular disease but rather as more susceptible than average to the hazards of relative over-nutrition and its interactions with other risk factors. The ageing participants in the long-term cohort studies[32] may help to identify aspects of adult lifestyle that mitigate the disadvantages of intrauterine and childhood deprivation. These mechanisms are important in the context of social inequalities as well as of ageing.

So far, much of what we know about extrinsic influences on ageing relates to unsurprising matters such as avoiding smoking and excess alcohol, maintaining a sensible diet and body weight and, perhaps most pervasively, regular adequate exercise. Observational studies suggest that exercise helps to establish and maintain bone and muscle strength, prevents vascular disease and may have other more general effects on wellbeing.[33] Randomised controlled trials of lifestyle modifications are unlikely to be widely applicable although trials have indicated that exercise can reduce falls in later life[34] and produce short-term increases in weight-bearing bone density.[35] Demonstrating that lifestyle changes could be beneficial in improving the pattern of ageing is, however, less difficult than persuading people to adopt them – health education improves knowledge but has little effect in changing behaviour. There is a research agenda for the social sciences in identifying the opportunities and incentives for optimal lifestyles that could inform a public health approach to an ageing society. Again, thinking needs to be radical and strategic. If disability in later life can be reduced by increasing physical exercise at all ages, this might be better achieved not by providing vouchers for fitness centres but by making our urban environments safer and more pleasant for walkers and cyclists.

Intrinsic ageing

Intrinsic ageing presents a biological enigma. The increase with time in entropy of living organisms cannot be dismissed as a trivial consequence of the second law of thermodynamics, for that law applies only to closed systems and biological organisms are open systems. Indeed, a capacity for self-repair has long been recognised as one of the properties of living organisms, and although individual organisms deteriorate with time the germplasm remains intact over innumerable generations.

It was suggested in the 19th century that ageing represented programmed obsolescence, conferring benefit on a species by removing the old to make way for the more adaptable young. One still hears such notions urged, but evolution cannot work that way; the units of selection are not species but genes and the individual organisms carrying them. More fundamentally, it is not necessary to invoke programmed death as a general phenomenon because, in the wild, death from natural causes is an inevitability. There are some cited examples of apparent programmed death; the most intriguing of which affects the female Octopus hummelincki in which rapid wasting and death normally follows reproduction but can be prevented by removal of the optic gland.[36] Other apparent instances, for example in Pacific salmon or the male marsupial mouse,[37] can be interpreted as selectively neutral side effects of basically adaptive reproductive behaviour.

Four groups of genes affect the pattern of our ageing. Some are deleterious genes that have their effects in later life and so are not eradicated by natural selection. Under natural conditions death is inevitable, and selective pressure on genes declines as a function of time after the onset of reproductive capacity.[38,39] Late onset deleterious genes can be invisible to evolution; of medical relevance are those for late onset neurological disorders including Alzheimer's and Huntington's disease.

The pattern of ageing experienced by individuals or tribes is also affected by genetic polymorphisms that are potentially accessible to selective pressure. Some will be 'pleiotropic' genes which have been selected because of benefits conferred in early life even though they may have deleterious effects at later ages.[40] They include the 'thrifty genes' already mentioned,[30] the haemoglobinopathies and other polymorphisms for which past or present selective advantage can be surmised. Other genes in this group include those determining blood pressure response to dietary sodium or the metabolism of tobacco smoke, whose evolutionary significance is less apparent but which affect individuals' interactions with their environments.

A third group of genes comprises those affecting ageing at a cellular and subcellular level and are thought to act by determining the efficiency of damage control. Damage arises from factors in the organism's internal and external environments including trauma, radiation, heat and chemical reactions. Unless controlled by processes of prevention, detection and repair or replacement, damage will accumulate and eventually prove fatal. Kirkwood's concept of the disposable soma provides the clearest model of how damage control affects the evolution of ageing and lifespan.[41] An organism has a limited intake of energy and other resources and natural selection will lead to its allocating these so as to maximise the survival of its genes into succeeding generations. The crucial balance is between reproduction rate and the investment in damage control that will determine ageing rate and longevity. Damage control, for example by protein turnover or chemical proofreading in replicating molecules, is expensive in energy. In a dangerous environment, where life will of necessity be short, the optimal strategy will be to invest in a high rate of reproduction rather than damage control. In a less dangerous environment it may be better for the organism to retard ageing, and while reproducing more slowly to develop strategies to ensure that a higher percentage of offspring survive to reproductive capacity. Such strategies include parental care and restricting breeding to times of year when offspring will have a plentiful food supply. Kirkwood's crucial insight was to show that in the case of intraspecific competition the investment in repair that provides the optimal evolutionary fitness will inevitably be at a level less than that necessary entirely to abolish ageing. During our evolution as a species we have greatly lengthened our maximum lifespan, compared with our close relatives the chimpanzees, but we have only retarded, not abolished, senescence.

A corollary of the evolutionary pressure towards maximal efficiency of resource allocation is that ageing will not be paced by any single process. Each body system that has energy requirements will evolve in step and will be tuned to the same overall lifespan. This can mislead those who seek a single underlying ageing process or 'biological clock'. The efficiency of repair of DNA damage in different species is correlated with lifespan,[42] for example, not because it is the rate-limiting factor in senescence, but simply because it could not be otherwise. Ageing can only be understood through models that are constrained by the co-evolution of cellular and subcellular mechanisms and their inter-actions. Kirkwood and Kowald[43] have developed such a model embodying the accumulation of defective mitochondria, the effects of aberrant proteins, free radical damage and protein turnover. This model fits a number of the features of instability observed during cellular ageing.

A comprehensive network model could predict where inter-ventions might retard cellular ageing. Meanwhile, there are two main lines of research aimed at modifying the rate of human age-ing. We are genetically so close to shorter lived primates that the number of genes that are involved in producing our longer life-span may be finite. One line of research therefore focuses on the identification of relevant genes and their mechanisms of action. Relevant genes are sought through homology with lower organisms and by a search for 'longevity assurance genes' that occur more often in the genomes of centenarians than in those of younger people. The second line of research seeks means of reducing damage load in general or on particular cellular components such as the mitochondria.[44] Damage from free radicals produced in mitochondrial metabolism, for example, might be achieved by increased antioxidant concentrations, or through reducing un-productive metabolism by food restriction. Caloric restriction prolongs lifespan in several species[45] but may not work by reducing free radical damage; in the species studied it may be another example of a metabolic switch prolonging survival by reducing reproduction rate. This capability would improve selective fitness by enabling an organism to survive times of privation to reproduce when food becomes more abundant. There is no evidence that the rate of ageing of Homo sapiens can be reduced by caloric restric-tion. The association of amenorrhoea with low body-weight does, however, suggest the existence of a mechanism for inhibiting reproduction during times of privation.

The fourth group of genes of geratological significance reflects the evolutionary history of Homo sapiens as a species. Primate species show three main forms of social organisation that select for characteristic morphological features.[46] In what we may designate as promiscuous societies males and females distribute their sexual favours widely; the sexes are typically of similar size and the males show a high ratio of testicular weight to body-weight. This is because of the need to produce large quantities of spermatozoa to compete with those of other males in the female genital tract. In the harem type of organisation a single male has sole rights to the breeding females around him and therefore can have smaller testes. Males are bigger than females as they have to compete for control of harems and the bigger males win. Also the females choose to join the harems of the bigger males since if the male is defeated in combat the victor may kill the offspring of his predecessor. Some primate species are monogamous and the sexes of equal size; the males show a range of testicular weights suggesting that they have evolved from one or other of the other two patterns (Fig 6). It is clear from our morphology that Homo sapiens is derived from a primate with a harem type of organisation like the gorilla. In the category of geratological curiosity is the phenomenon of hair greying. The dominant male gorilla in a harem develops the striking appearance of a 'silverback' and may secure some advantage from thus signalling his advancing years. Young male gorillas will not lightly challenge a harem owner who demonstrably has been around long enough to have seen off plenty of young pretenders like them before. To females, the silver back indicates that its owner is a good survivor and likely to contribute good genes to their progeny. A preference of females for older mates has been documented elsewhere, for example in

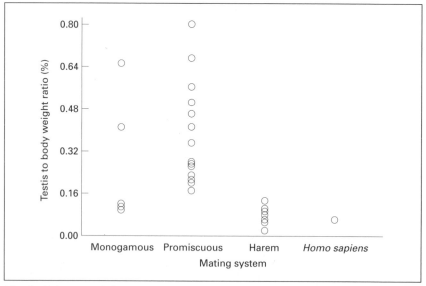

Fig 6. *Primate social organisation and ratio of testis to body weight.* Data from Harcourt *et al*[46]

the cactus finch, the males of which grow darker with each season they survive – the females mate preferentially with darker males.[47] The supposed attractiveness of greying temples in men seems the sole remnant of this influence on sexual selection in Homo sapiens.

The biological superiority of the human female

With this background we are closer to being able to account for the paradox that women outlive men but are more likely to be disabled in later life. It began in the primal harem: there females have less opportunity for reproduction than the male and so are under more selective pressure to live longer to contribute more offspring to the next generation. This form of selective pressure would have been acting before the evolution of the menopause. The females of our ancestor species would have shown the universal pattern of reproductive capability in higher animals that as their age increased they would be less likely to produce viable offspring and more likely to die in the attempt. The menopause is thought to have arisen at a time when one of our ancestral groups had developed a cumulative culture based on speech, or a forerunner of speech, and had a family-based form of social organisation. In such circumstances there could come a time in the lives of women when in terms of getting their genes into later generations it would be better to give up increasingly dangerous and unsuccessful attempts to produce children of their own, even though each would contain 50% of their genes, and instead to contribute to the survival of their grandchildren, each of which carries 25% of their genes. We may further postulate that this happened at the same time that maximum lifespan of the species was lengthening under the pressure of a safer environment as predicted by Kirkwood. As the maximum lifespan of the female lengthened to beyond a hundred years the lifespan of the ovary remained at 50 because there was no selective advantage in prolonging it. This 'grandmother hypothesis' is sometimes attacked on the grounds that in primitive societies no one would have lived beyond the age of 50 and so selective pressure could not have operated above that age. This assertion is based on the estimation of ages at death of skeletons found archaeologically and methods are very imprecise.[48] Better estimates of conditions among our hunter–gatherer ancestors come from studies of such societies that have survived to the present. Three studies have found that around 20% of people survive to the age of 60 and 10% to 70.[49]

The second cause of greater longevity of women probably lay in the neolithic era when hunter-gatherer cultures gave way to farming of fields and livestock. The survival of a tribe became dependent on a warrior caste to defend its crops and stocks and if these failed to steal someone else's. The warrior caste would have been composed of the larger males and would have had prior claim on food resources. Women would be regarded as disposable chattels partly because of contemporary understanding of genetics based on an agricultural model: the male produced the seed of the next generation and the female was merely the ground in which the seed grew. This idea can be found in one reading of Aristotle although he may not have held consistently to this view. If women were considered merely seedbeds, men would not have worried about breeding from the women of a defeated or inferior tribe; if one's own tribe fell short of women one stole someone else's. Plutarch's tale of Romulus's abduction of the Sabine women may have originated in a folk memory of such an event. The low priority of women in food distribution would favour adaptations to undernutrition such as enhanced immune protection against infectious diseases at the expense of body size. When women came to live with men on more equal terms in later centuries their biological superiority emerged. Data are unreliable but the greater longevity of women seems to be an historically recent phenomenon.

Extrinsic factors in the 20th century provide a third source of female superiority. This can be seen in a plot of sex ratios of death rates against age (Fig 7). In the 19th century we can see the greater vulnerability of male infants to infectious disease and the effects of discrimination and childbirth in younger adult women. In the early years of this century the sex ratios were fairly constant across the lifespan at 1.1. Since then there has been a dramatic increase in male/female mortality ratios in young adult and late middle life. The younger of the two peaks is due to violent deaths and disappears if these are excluded from the calculations. The later peak, which is much more important in terms of numbers of deaths, is to a large extent attributable to smoking related diseases. Speculatively we might take the situation in 1911 as our best approximation to the intrinsic superiority of the female. This amounted to about 3.8 years in life expectancy at birth, while the additional 2.2 years women have acquired in this century are due to extrinsic factors.

The higher risk of disability among women in later life is also partly attributable to our evolutionary history. The primal harem

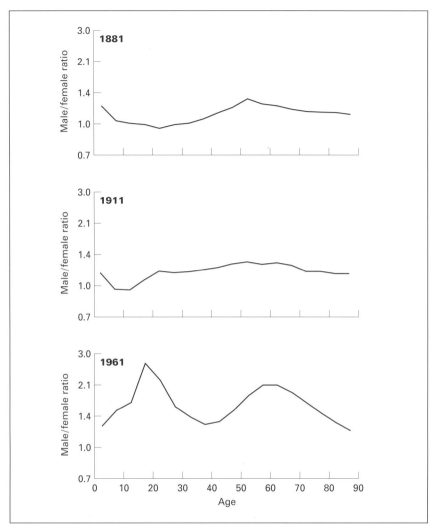

Fig 7. *Male to female ratio of age-specific mortality rates in England: 1881–90, 1911 and 1961*

led to males being bigger than females with more bone and muscle at maturity. Both sexes lose muscle and strength with time and by the time they are in their 80s most women do not have enough muscle left to rise from a chair without using their arms[50]. This difference in muscle strength is probably the single most important contributor to the high levels of disability in women in later life. Whether it could be overcome by more exercise throughout life is an important issue unlikely to be resolvable by randomised controlled trials.

The future

The public health response to the ageing population is to adjust the environment and lifestyle of a nation to produce the best overall outcome, given the genetic propensities of the population. Table 1 presents the grounds for hoping that this will achieve the geratological aim of lengthening life but shortening disability. Among women, on whom the major burden of disability falls, Table 1 suggests that the older a woman is while still independent, the shorter the period of disability she can expect before death. There is an underlying epidemiological logic here, since as a result of the loss of adaptability – the characteristic feature of ageing – the later the onset of a potentially disabling disease such as stroke, the more likely it is to prove fatal. This provides the rationale for a policy of postponement as prevention. Although we do not know what is happening in the UK, recent data from the USA are encouraging in showing that the prevalence of disability at later ages has been falling while average lifespan has been increasing.[51] This seems to have come about not because of improvements in medical care, nor because of increased mortality among the disabled, but because successive generations of older people are showing a healthier pattern of ageing. This is what one would expect from a successful policy of postponement as prevention instituted as a public health measure. In the longer term we might learn how to apply the principle at an individual level. This might be achieved by modifying the action of genes; alternatively, citizens might learn to live a personally prescribed lifestyle to match their individual genotype and the state of their metabolic switches. Ethicists might worry over whether we should receive this prescription from our general practitioners or our insurance brokers.

We can hope that postponement as prevention would reduce healthcare costs. We cannot be sure, however, because the nature of disability as well as its average duration may change with age. Care for older people with dementia could be more expensive than for younger people with stroke. So far little work has been done on predicting the effects of 'substitute morbidity' arising as causes of disability and death change over time.[52] This is a particular concern in relation to research on intrinsic ageing which, if successful, will lengthen maximum lifespan but have unpredictable effects on the incidence and duration of disability. We can recognise the political difficulties that might arise if lengthening the lives of people, even with a reduction in the average time spent in a disabled state, increased their lifetime costs of health care.

It is important that we do not let fears of what might be prevent our exploration of what could be. The ageing of populations is not a transient epidemic that will pass; it is a permanent change in the structure of society to which society and individuals must adapt. The new political configuration in Europe offers us wider opportunities than we have ever enjoyed for research into the intrinsic and extrinsic causes and mechanisms of ageing, and into the design and funding of health and social services. The chief impediment, as I have hinted, is likely to be political paralysis. The need for a long-term view, the possibility of being confronted with difficult decisions, including the issue of inter-generational inequities in funding, make it unlikely that government will provide the leadership and vision necessary to prepare the nation for the challenges to come. The leadership will have to come from within the ranks of the knowledgeable and socially responsible citizenry. Therein the medical profession is pre-eminent, and what better principle to guide us than 'a correct compassion, that performs its love'.

References

1 Herringham W. William Harvey at St Bartholomew's. *St Bartholomew's Hospital Journal* 1928; **35**: 13–6.
2 Kirkup, J. A correct compassion. In:*A correct compassion and other poems.* Oxford: Oxford University Press, 1952.
3 World Health Organisation Scientific Group on the Epidemiology of Ageing. *The uses of epidemiology in the study of the elderly. Technical Report Series No 706.* Geneva: World Health Organisation, 1984.
4 Grimley Evans J. Healthy active life expectancy (HALE) as an index of effectiveness of health and social services for elderly people. *Age Ageing* 1993; **22**: 297–301.
5 Dunnell K. Population review: 2. Are we healthier? In: *Population Trends 82.* London: HMSO, 1995: 12–8.
6 Katz S, Branch LG, Bransom MH, Papidero JA, *et al.* Active life expectancy. *New England Journal of Medicine* 1983; **309**: 1218–24.
7 van de Water HPA, Boshuizen HC, Perenboom RJN. Health expectancy in the Netherlands 1983–1990. *European Journal of Public Health* 1996; **6**: 21–8.
8 Kemper P, Murtaugh CM. Lifetime use of nursing home care. *New England Journal of Medicine* 1991; **324**: 595–600.
9 Office of Population Censuses and Surveys Social Survey Division. Martin J, Meltzer H, Elliot D. *OPCS surveys of disability in Great Britain Report 1. The prevalence of disability among adults.* London: HMSO, 1988.
10 Government Actuary. *National population projections 1994-based.* London: HMSO, 1996.
11 Laing W, Hall M. *Agenda for health 1991. The challenges of ageing.* London: Association of the British Pharmaceutical Industry, 1991.

12 Nuttall SR, Blackwood RJL, Bussell BMH, Cliff JP, *et al.* Financing long-term care in Great Britain. *Journal of the Institute of Actuaries* 1994; **121**: 1–53.

13 Callahan D. *Setting limits. Medical goals in an ageing society.* New York: Simon and Schuster, 1987.

14 Jahnigen DW, Binstock RH. Economic and clinical realities: health care for elderly people. In: Binstock RH, Post SG (eds). *Too old for health care? Controversies in medicine, law, economics and ethics.* Baltimore: The Johns Hopkins University Press, 1991: 13–43.

15 Thomson D. Generations, justice and the future of collective action. In: Laslett P, Fishkin JS (eds). *Justice between age groups and generations.* London: Yale University Press, 1992: 206–35.

16 Williams A. Rationing health care by age: the case for. *British Medical Journal* 1997; **314**: 8–9.

17 Grimley Evans J. Rationing health care by age: the case against. *British Medical Journal* 1997; **314**: 11–12.

18 Mill JS. *On liberty.* London: John W Parker and Son, West Strand, 1859.

19 Browne JP, O'Boyle CA, McGee HM, Joyce CR, *et al.* Individual quality of life in the healthy elderly. *Quality of Life Research* 1994; **3**: 235–44.

20 Ouslander JG, Tymchuk AJ, Rahbar B. Health care decisions among elderly long-term care residents and their potential proxies. *Archives of Internal Medicine* 1989; **149**: 1367–72.

21 Seckler AB, Meier DE, Mulvihill M, Cammer Paris BE. Substituted judgement: how accurate are proxy predictions? *Annals of Internal Medicine* 1991; **115**: 92–8.

22 Grimley Evans J. Hospital care for the elderly. In: Shegog REA (ed). *The impending crisis of old age.* London: Nuffield Provincial Hospitals Trust, 1981: 133–46.

23 Rubenstein LZ. The efficacy of geriatric assessment programmes. In: Kane RL, Grimley Evans J, Macfadyen D (eds). *Improving the health of older people. A world view.* Oxford: Oxford University Press, 1990: 417–39.

24 Prior IAM, Grimley Evans J, Davidson F, Lindsay M. Sodium intake and blood pressure in two Polynesian populations. *New England Journal of Medicine* 1968; **279**: 515–20.

25 Goycoolea MV, Goycoolea HG, Rodriguez LG, Martinez GC, *et al.* Effect of life in industrialised societies on hearing in natives of Easter Island. *Laryngoscope* 1986; **96**: 1391–6.

26 Grimley Evans J, Seagroatt V, Goldacre MJ. Secular trends in proximal femoral fracture, Oxford Record Linkage Study area and England 1968–86. *Journal of Epidemiology and Community Health* 1997; **51**: 424–9.

27 Barker DJP. The fetal origins of diseases in old age. *European Journal of Clinical Nutrition* 1992; **46 (Suppl 3)**: S3–S9.

28 Devlin B, Daniels M, Roeder K. The heritability of IQ. *Nature* 1997; **388**: 468–71.

29 Grimley Evans J. Metabolic switches in ageing. *Age and Ageing* 1993; **22**: 79–81.

30 Neel JV. A 'thrifty' genotype rendered detrimental by progress? *American Journal of Human Genetics* 1962; **14**: 353–161.

31 McKeigue PM, Shah B, Marmot MG. Relation of central obesity and

insulin resistance with high diabetes prevalence and cardiovascular risk in South Asians. *Lancet* 1991; **337**: 382–6.

32   Wadsworth MEJ, Cripps HA, Midwinter RA, Colley JRT. Blood pressure at age 36 years and social and familial factors, cigarette smoking and body mass in a national birth cohort. *British Medical Journal* 1985; **291**: 1534–8.

33   Curfman CD. The health benefits of exercise. A critical reappraisal. *New England Journal of Medicine* 1993; **328**: 574–6.

34   Province MA, Hadley EC, Hornbrook MC, Lipsitz LA, *et al.* The effects of exercise on falls in elderly patients. A preplanned meta-analysis of the FICSIT trials. *Journal of the American Medical Association* 1995; **273**: 1341–7.

35   Brooke-Wavell K, Jones PRM, Hardman AE. Brisk walking reduces calcaneal bone loss in post-menopausal women. *Clinical Science* 1996; **92**: 75–80.

36   Wodinsky J. Hormonal inhibition of feeding and death in Octopus. Control by optic gland secretion. *Science* 1977; **198**: 948–51.

37   Diamond JM. Big-bang reproduction and ageing in male marsupial mice. *Nature* 1982; **298**: 115–6.

38   Medawar P. *An unsolved problem in biology*, London: Lewis, 1952.

39   Hamilton WD. The moulding of senescence by natural selection. *Journal of Theoretical Biology* 1966; **12**: 12–45.

40   Williams GC. Pleiotropy, natural selection and the evolution of senescence. *Evolution* 1957; **11**: 398–411.

41   Kirkwood TBL, Rose MR. Evolution of senescence: late survival sacrificed for reproduction. *Philosophical Transactions of the Royal Society Series B* 1991; **332**: 15–24.

42   Hart RW, Setlow RB. Correlation between deoxyribonucleic acid excision repair and life-span in a number of mammalian species. *Proceedings of the National Academy of Science* 1974; **71**: 2169–73.

43   Kirkwood TBL, Kowald A. Network theory of ageing. *Experimental Gerontology* 1997; **32**: 395–9.

44   Shigenaga MK, Hagen TM, Ames BN. Oxidative damage and mitochondrial decay in aging. *Proceedings of the National Academy of Science* 1994; **91**: 10771–8.

45   Masoro EJ. Dietary restriction and aging. *Journal of American Geriatric Society* 1993; **41**: 994–9.

46   Harcourt AH, Harvey PH, Larson SG, Short RV. Testis weight, body weight and breeding system in primates. *Nature* 1981; **293**: 55–7.

47   Grant BR, Grant PR. Mate choice in Darwin's finches. *Biological Journal of the Linnean Society* 1987; **32**: 247–70.

48   Mollesen TI. Skeletal age and palaeodemography. In: Bittles AH, Collins KJ (eds). *The biology of human ageing*. Cambridge: Cambridge University Press, 1986: 95–118.

49   Hill K, Hurtado M. The evolution of premature reproductive senescence and menopause in human females: an evaluation of the 'grandmother hypothesis'. *Human Nature* 1991; **2**: 313–50.

50   Young A. Exercise physiology in geriatric practice. *Acta Medica Scandinavia* 1986; **Suppl 711**: 227–32.

51   Manton KG, Corder L, Stallard E. Chronic disability trends in elderly United States populations: 1982–1994. *Proceedings of the National Academy of Science* 1997; **94**: 2593–8.

52 van de Water HPA, van Vliet HA, Boshuizen HC. *The impact of 'substitute morbidity and mortality' on public health policy.* Leiden: TNO Prevention and Health Division Public Health and Prevention, 1995.